BEYOND REDEMPTION

JESSE LORENZO

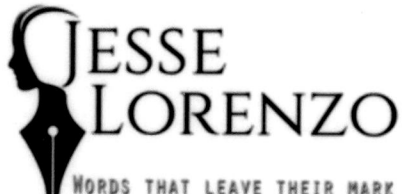

JESSE LORENZO

WORDS THAT LEAVE THEIR MARK

TABLE OF CONTENTS

DEDICATION

To my three beautiful daughters,
Jazlyn, Veronica, and Marcela:
Dream big and reach for the stars.
Mommy loves you.

BEYOND
REDEMPTION

PROLOGUE

A soft summer breeze drifted inside the open second-story window, carrying with it the calming scent of the salty sea air. Gulls cawed their claim on the Harbor as they coasted high above the pier. Ellora sat on her padded window seat, gazing through her sheer curtains as they danced with the wind. They moved with the rhythm of the tide, gently fanning her face.

She watched the hustle of the townies as they made good work of a clear, beautiful day, loading and docking their fishing boats and gear. As they went about their lives, she imagined that she could do the same... and move on with hers. Ellora rose from her peaceful place when hunger pains growled irritably in her empty stomach.

The dazed girl aimlessly lumbered around her kitchenette, searching for something to stifle her appetite. Mindlessly gathering an array of random food choices, she placed the items on her tiny table. Reaching into the drawer, she retrieved a knife to spread mustard on her plain sandwich. Ellora held the utensil in her hands, turning it around in her grasp several times. Sunlight that splashed in through her open window bounced off the reflective surface of the sleek metal and cast an iridescent rainbow on her solemn face. A reoccurring nightmare that she was unable to shake flashed behind her eyes, of a monster trying to take her life.

It had been a few weeks since Ellora was assaulted by the man she feared most in the world. Giddeon still remained in the jailhouse located in the center of town, but Detective Antonelli assured her that he was doing everything he could to transfer him out of Portree and back to the States.

The terrifying thought of her attacker being housed so close to where she lived, set her nerves on edge. She just didn't feel safe with him only walking distance away. Just like any other powerful monster, he seemed capable of breaking free from his prison. Ellora lived in a constant state of fear that he could still get to her, that it was only a matter of time before he would.

This fear had taken control of her life, forcing her to become a prisoner as well. Ellora became incredibly anxious when alone in her self-made fortress, and at the same time, loud noisy crowds made her jumpy and nervous. She couldn't seem to find solace in any given situation. It was a double-edged sword that left her confined to her second floor safe haven. Her emotional handicap kept her away from Grady's Pub downstairs on most busy nights, locked away in her room.

Deep down, she knew her behavior made those who cared about her extremely worried for her mental stability. Everyone except, of course, Behr. He, more than anyone else, understood what she was going through. Behr had witnessed her attack firsthand, and lived through a close call of his own when he fought the devil himself... and won. If she thought of him as overprotective before, that was nothing compared to how he acted now.

Ellora couldn't step foot into a room without Behr giving it a swift once-over first. At night, he checked every room, behind every door, and in every nook and cranny. He'd even go as far as checking under her bed to make sure his love would be safe, before kissing her goodnight.

Once the sun brightened the pier with rich shades of orange that glistened on the water's surface at sunrise, Behr would wake her with the delicious smell of breakfast. This had become their routine. He'd hardly ever left her side since the attack, and she didn't mind in the least. Ellora wanted him there, right by her side, while she tried her best to pick up the pieces of her life.

Like always, Behr understood what she needed and tried his best to give it to her so that they could finally move on with their lives—time, patience, and love. Most importantly, she wanted to be happy... to live a normal life and enjoy every moment of it without any fear. It warmed her heart to think about the future. Each and every glimpse of it had Behr standing right beside her. She had fallen so hard for him over the course of a few months.

Stuck in the blissful daydreams of the chivalrous man she loved, Ellora hadn't heard the door to her flat open, or the figure approaching from behind her. When a heavy hand came down on her shoulder, she jumped a good foot off the ground. A strangled shriek scratched her throat as she choked on her scream. Ellora spilled all the food she had laid out while preparing her lunch, scattering the condiments onto the parched wooden floors.

Strong arms wrapped around her tiny waist in a firm grip. Without a moment's pause, he spoke. "It's a'right, love. It's just me. I came as soon as my tour 'round the Isle was completed. I dinnae mean to startle ya." Kissing her throbbing temple, helplessness welled up inside him as her trembling frame sagged against him in relief. He wished he could make all of her fears disappear once and for all.

Behr tightened his arms around the frightened girl, giving her the reassuring support she needed. "I'm sorry, Lor."

"It's okay, Behr. I'm… I'm okay. I just keep forgetting that I gave you a key, and my mind wasn't present when you walked in. Otherwise, I'm sure I would've heard you."

The quiet man nodded against her cheek, abrading it with his day old stubble. "I came by to let ya know that I received word that *he* is leaving tomorrow. That bastard will never come anywhere near ya again."

Ellora filled her lungs with a long, deep breath of

renewed relief. When she blew it out, the enormous weight that was dragging her down had been removed from her spirit. She'd suffered from the crushing burden of fear and anxiety for so long that she had grown accustomed to the extra baggage she carried around. Now... finally, it had been released, and she felt as weightless as the air she pulled in.

Turning into Behr's protective embrace, she weaved her arms around his neck, running her fingers through his thick hair. "That's the best news I've gotten in weeks." The enormous man struck her with a smile that could have stadiums full of women swooning at the sight.

"Aye, that's because no one's told you of the little *incident* that happened to me last week."

Ellora giggled softly, lifting a curious brow, waiting for him to spill his guts.

"My pants got caught on a loose divot on the Ferry while I was giving her a good wash, and split right along the rear seam, all the way down. In front of all the world. Gave the whole pier an eyeful of my arse, I did."

Behr delighted in the beautiful sound of her whole-hearted laughter as it shook her tiny frame against his chest. He hadn't heard her laugh in a long while, and that in itself killed him.

"Oh, I'm *really* sorry I missed *that*! Did you at least get any good tips from the tourists for the free show?"

"Aye. Bought me a new pair o' pants with it. Good thing I decided to wear underwear that day."

Ellora threw her head back and laughed harder, slapping him playfully. "You would've gotten better tips, Captain Buchanan, had you forgotten. Lesson learned."

"Sit down, my love, and let me prepare your lunch. We can celebrate starting over."

Ellora loved the sound of that. After all, she couldn't live in this tiny room, hidden away, forever. The thought of finally starting her life over, with Behr by her side, was definitely something worth celebrating. Lifting the glass he had poured for her, she announced, "To starting a new life... together."

She couldn't wait to find out what the future held for them.

Portree Harbor:
Municipal Jailhouse

iddeon had been dumped into this tiny whole in the wall hours ago. It just so happened to be a typical run of the mill 'get 'em talkin' interrogation room. You've seen one, you've seen them all. Nine-by-twelve, low drop ceiling with yellow flickering florescent lights, beckoning you into madness as it pulsated harshly inside the cramped space. The longer Giddeon sat, the further his mind succumbed to the excruciating sting of the unforgiving light. A growing migraine sliced through his ability to concentrate, like thousands of glass shards cutting through the sensitive areas of his brain. All this was intentional.

Giddeon rubbed at his eyes with his iron clad hands, the cuffs only allowing a few inches of leeway as they were attached to the stainless steel table in the center of the room. There were two chairs. His, a small, metal, extremely uncomfortable chair. Its hard surface left him numb from the waist down after hours of sitting in one spot. The legs were all uneven, creating an awkward tilt, and the metal spokes left deep imprints onto his back. The other chair, a luxuriously padded, ergonomic rocker on wheels. Also very intentional. It was all a mental game they loved to play.

Slate grey tiles lined the floor, and an equally dreary color blandly covered the walls. One steel door was across the room from him and a two-way mirror behind him. Nothing else. The room stayed subzero in temperature, due to the air conditioner blowing at full blast. It left him shivering uncontrollably in his metal chair.

Giddeon fixated on every minute detail of the ice box of a room. Countless suspects had been present in this same room, sweating out their guilt. That was evident by the smell that lingered in the air. Like an old gym locker room mixed with the unmistakable stench of stale cigarettes.

Voices and footsteps pulled his idle mind back to the here and now. Detective Antonelli leisurely walked in with a thick accordion folder under one arm, and two steaming Styrofoam cups. One in each hand. He set them down carefully and quietly lowered himself into the chair, rocking methodically... back and forth, testing its comfort. Several tense moments ticked by as the men stared at one another, sizing each other up.

Giddeon's eyes narrowed on his target, inspecting his appearance. The detective's nose was braced, bandaged, and crooked. Dry blood coated the inside of his nostrils, and fresh bruises painted his eyes black and blue. He looked rough. A smile tugged at the prisoner's lips at the sight of him. The same knowing smirk was mirrored on the detective's face.

"Did the big guy get you, too, Detective?" Dominick forced out a painful sounding chuckle as he slid the steaming black coffee in Giddeon's direction. He silently thanked God for simple pleasures such as this.

"Hey, at least we can tell people we fought a bear and lived to tell about it, right?" Giddeon nodded, agreeing with him. The man who left both men battered and broken, coincidentally named Behr, was the greatest adversary and the finest fight he'd had in years. As a fighter, he'd gained an enormous respect for the man.

Behr was Giddeon's polar opposite. He had courage, love, and a light within him, all things the twisted man didn't possess but desperately wished he did. One could just look at the large man and see it pouring out as he bravely fought to rescue the woman he loved. Rescue her from Giddeon.

A manic laugh belted out of him, a delightfully painful jolt ebbing through his damaged jaw. The harsh throbbing coursed through all his extremities, like the powerful sting from a scorpion's strike. It awakened a dark desire deep inside him. Giddeon laughed harder, and quickly came to the conclusion soon after that his jaw was either seriously cracked or dislocated.

Along with that injury, he also suffered a swollen-shut left eye, a split wide open cheek, and a skillfully stitched up shoulder. All of which were inflicted by the powerful hands of Behr. The pain that followed had him riding a beautiful never ending high. He had denied any pain medication, and insisted on being stitched up without a numbing agent.

The throbbing ebbed and pulsed through his badly beaten body. It was a reminder that he was alive... human. Giddeon hadn't been this badly beaten since... since... No! He wouldn't let his mind wander there. Not in front of the detective. Shaking his head in order to snap himself out of the dangerous thought that still played around in his head, he looked at the detective.

Dominick nodded his head in the direction of the cuffed man, taking stock of his numerous injuries. "He almost killed you."

Giddeon ignored his truthful statement and addressed his earlier comment about Behr. "Yup, surviving a Behr attack is definitely a good story to be told. What'd you do to piss him off, anyway?" The detective leaned far back in his chair, eyeing him thoughtfully. Giddeon didn't like *that* look—the look of pity. His humor and patience slipped away as he glared at him, wishing his hands weren't cuffed so that he could wipe *that* look right off his face.

Dominick snapped out of his thoughts, shook his head, and laughed. He gingerly grasped the bridge of his cracked nose. "I guess he didn't like the way I was looking at his girl in the pub... kinda like the way you're not liking the way I'm looking at you. Maybe I'll use this injury as an excuse to get a new face. You think workers comp will cover facial reconstruction under my insurance?" he joked, lightening up the mounting tension. It died down quickly, and they both laughed at his expense. This fucker was funny.

"I highly doubt Dalton will give that the green light, since you're still technically working for him, right?"

Their laughter awkwardly died down. "I think it's safe to say that, after this stunt, I've quit. And I'm probably fired, anyway."

Silence stretched out, leaving the conversation at an uncomfortable stand still. Giddeon's cuffed hands, attached to the bolted down table, picked at the dried up blood and debris under his ridged nails. "Well..." Giddeon paused, shaking off the calculated pleasantries, and glared at him, unblinking, directly in the eyes.

The detective's demeanor changed, as well, turning serious, and he stared right back at the cuffed man, undaunted by his silent threat. "Dalton turned his back on you, didn't he?"

Anger burned deep in the pit of the dark man's stomach. He stiffly nodded... just once. "He did." The beast stirred within him, looking to exact his revenge. A familiar itch, desperately needing to be scratched, surfaced, making his skin crawl. Like a junkie anticipating his next fix, Giddeon wanted to satisfy his addiction. He needed to hurt someone, and it didn't matter who.

Thoughts swirled in his head of all he'd done for Dalton, all the vile things he'd made him do, pulling him deeper and deeper into a soulless void. These thoughts awakened a deep seated need to collect his blood, as hate and vengeance roused a powerful rage inside him. The overwhelming feeling stole away his breath. He closed his eyes, imagining Dalton pleading for his pathetic life as Giddeon squeezed his carotid tighter and tighter. He longed to hear the gurgling noises escaping the lips of his victim as he fought to pull air into his seizing lungs.

A ghost of a smile danced across Giddeon's lips as he longed for the day he could see Dalton's all-consuming fear paralyze him... in person. Glaring into his cold eyes, he wanted nothing more than to take his power and control from him... as he took his life. This fantasy would keep Giddeon moving forward until the day he could finally douse the hungry beast that lay waiting. Waiting for the day he could squeeze the betrayal right out of Dalton.

Scalding hot sensations abruptly brought the disturbed man back to reality as the detective snatched the now crushed cup from his clenched fists. The coffee burned a magnificent trail down his hands and wrists, dripping onto the table. The images of Dalton's bloodshot eyes clouding over as death claimed him still hovered in his consciousness.

Dominick handed him a napkin to clean himself off

with.

"That betrayal leaves a bitter aftertaste, doesn't it?"

Giddeon gritted his teeth, biting down so hard he was surprised his teeth didn't chip under the punishing pressure. "I'm going to fucking kill him."

The detective leaned across the table. Serious determination was written all over his face. "You and me both. I want Dalton. I know he's behind it all, and I don't care what I have to do. I'm taking him down."

Giddeon liked the thought of that. "I think this is what you call meeting on common ground, Detective. We both want the same things for different reasons."

A confident smile crept across Dominick's face as he nodded in agreement.

"I'm taking you back to the States with me, where you'll be classified as my Criminal Informant. Give me everything I need to take down Dalton, and I will make sure the prosecutor in your case is lenient with your situation. If you cooperate fully, I will be in your corner. It's a win-win. You help me... I help you. Deal?"

"I don't deserve leniency! And I don't fucking deserve your mercy!" Giddeon snapped, growling out his fury, as spit flew out of his salivating mouth. "It's going to take a lot more than a cop or a twisted fucked-up person like me to bring him down. Don't you understand? He has more people in his pocket than you can possibly imagine. Even agents in *your* department, Detective."

Dominick slammed his fists on the stainless steel table. Standing, he shouted back, "I'm not in his pocket! Are you? You his little pocket puppet? Are you afraid of going up against him? Well, I'm not! I've got nothing to lose, and I'm sure as shit not stopping until his ass is rotting in a six-by-eight shithole. Do you understand me? No one's going to stand in my way."

Giddeon sat watching the detective freak the hell out, admiring his tenacity. He realized then that they were two sides to the same coin, both driven by an obsessive need to find the same man. He had to respect that. "Are you ready to go down this road, Detective? Are you ready to lose your career... your life? Because that's exactly what Dalton will go after."

"You're damn fucking right, I am." Dominick pointed his meaty finger in his face.

"Why are you pushing this so hard? I'm not the sort of person to be trusted. You don't know me. You don't know what I've done, or what I'm capable of."

The detective got up and paced the room, never taking his eyes off the dark, cuffed man. An odd expression appeared on his face. It twisted at Giddeon's gut as warning bells sounded off inside his head. Halting his pacing, Dominick seemingly came to some kind of decision as he walked back over to the table with purpose. The detective tapped the cold table with his finger. "Obviously, we ran your prints..." Grabbing the envelope, he reached inside and let out a deep breath, as if what he was about to reveal inside was difficult to bring up.

Giddeon knew that whatever was in there, was about to change *everything*. Slowly, the detective pulled out a file as thick as a novel, dropping it on the table. The smooth, stainless steel surface had them skittering across its length. Several photos landed directly in front of Giddeon. His stomach bottomed out.

"I know who you are... Giddeon Cane. You have been missing for quite some time." Dominick's voice sounded distant to Giddeon's ears, and he felt the blood slowly drain from his face. He stared blankly, unable to blink, at a photograph of his deceased parents, embracing outside their old brownstone. The other photograph, a coroner's photo of their cold, stiff bodies on a metal slab. They stared hauntingly back up at him. His surroundings changed, turning surreal, like Giddeon was standing outside of himself looking in. Bile rose up and threatened to exit. He swallowed forcefully, attempting to hold the growing knot at bay. His vision tunneled as he zeroed in on the photo of his parents.

The longer he stared, the more he slipped into a memory he'd kept buried in the depths of his mind, long forgotten. "I've got a good idea of exactly *what* you've been through, Giddeon."

Giddeon was taken back to the tiny townhome he grew up in. *He could still smell the lemon scented cleaner his mom used to polish the hardwood floors and tables. It was her scheduled weekend cleaning ritual. A young Giddeon skipped up the stone steps with his dad. They were practicing hitting the bag and sparring with a few other members at the local gym. His father was a very strong fighter, a two time golden gloves winner. Giddeon loved watching him in the ring. It became their weekend father-son bonding time. At the very young age of six, he was starting to show him proper stance, the use of a well-placed jab, and how to mix up his combinations.*

They would come home after a few hours to be greeted with the fresh lemon scent. On one particular day, Giddeon's mother had the radio on so loud she didn't hear them come in. His dad did his best to sneak up on her stealthily. He wrapped his arms around her waist and brought her to him quickly, achieving his intended goal... She jumped a good foot off the ground, startled by his silent approach. His mother giggled playfully as she turned to face him. Slapping him several times was his punishment for her racing heart.

Dad ran down the narrow hallway and into the cramped bathroom to avoid her stinging slaps as she gave chase after him. Little Giddeon ran after them as usual, entertained by their playful banter. As Mom cornered him, she turned the water faucet on full blast, splashing her husband with cold water. She accused him of smelling like a sweaty skunk and needing a bath. Her laughter came out breathlessly as she cupped the water, splashing Dad over and over. She compared the drenched man to a bristly ape that desperately needed a shave.

Dad lunged at her, containing her squiggling form in his strong unwavering arms. "All right, honey, pass the shaving cream, will ya." He slowly reached over, snatching up the cream, while Mom bucked and squealed, knowing full well his intensions. He doused his mother like a chef coating a cake with frosting. Shaving cream splattered everywhere. Their laughter and loving playfulness was forever etched in Giddeon's heart as he watched them from the doorway.

Just as quick as that memory flashed at him, it soon morphed into the horrific scene he witnessed not too long after. Giddeon frozen in place. Standing over their lifeless, cold bodies lying on the gritty family room floor. Their blood pooled in a large, stagnant puddle all around them. Their eyes wide open, but unseeing. The smells of sweat, fear, copper, and the faint lemon scent hung thickly in the humid summer air. The only noise was of the flies buzzing around the still forms of their decaying bodies.

All he could do was stand and stare. The feeling of petrified helplessness kept him frozen on the spot. Too afraid to move. Too afraid to utter a sound.

A devastating, grief-stricken sorrow crippled him. Giddeon crumpled up inside himself in painful agony. The hollowness inside of him was too heavy to bear as the old wounds were ripped wide opened. An unfamiliar haunting voice came ripping out of the depths of his blackened soul as he screamed out. The disturbing sound eerily echoed around the small empty room. Giddeon's face was wet with grieving tears he wasn't aware he had shed.

Giddeon was shaken out of his hellish nightmare, with the ghostly images of his parents' dead bodies and the horrid smell that burned his eyes and nose, so many years ago, still at the forefront of his vision.

Dominick violently shook him back to himself. Grateful that he pulled him out of the hell he tried so hard to bury, he was astonished that his black heart was still able to break after all this time.

That feeling was worse than any torture he had ever withstood. Worse than dying. That, at least, would be a gift. In that moment, Giddeon silently vowed to avenge their deaths. It was finally time. No more meaningless attacks, no more violent acts that never quenched his need for justice. He would help the detective and use him to find the men who murdered his parents. He didn't care what happened to him. The time had come... they deserved closure. Giddeon needed closure.

"Yes, I will help you, Detective. Whatever it takes, I'm in with you all the way. On one condition..." The detective lifted a questioning brow so Giddeon pressed on. "Help me find the men who murdered my parents. Re-open the case. That's all I want. Don't worry about trying to help or save me. I'm beyond help now. That's it. Take it or leave it."

Dominick reached over the table, extending his hand to be shook. "I would've helped you out with that anyway, now that I know who you are. You've got a deal." Giddeon reached as far as his cuffs would allow, grasping his hand and giving it a firm shake. Dominick turned, making his way out the door. "We leave in about two weeks. I just have to sign off and clear everything here. Sit tight in the meantime, and try not to get yourself in trouble with the Scottish authorities… or they will never let you leave."

Once the heavy door clicked shut, Giddeon took all his aggression out on the table in front of him, having no other way to release all his pent up feelings of anger, fear, helplessness, and grief. Giddeon's knuckles cracked wide open after a dozen or so strikes. His blood streaked across the otherwise clean surface.

Just like that, Giddeon's motive switched from an addictive need to inflict pain on others, to a desperate need for justice and revenge.

And he wouldn't stop until he got it.

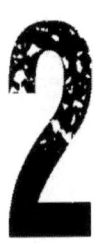

Portree Harbor,
Isle of Skye

things pretty much went back to normal after Detective Antonelli took Giddeon back to the States with him. Business as usual. Ellora was finally able to breathe easy, knowing he was in custody and as far away from Portree Harbor as possible. Her nightmares had been few and far between. She guessed that confronting him face-to-face and fighting him helped to overcome her greatest fears. He wasn't untouchable. He wasn't some unstoppable monster. He was just a man. He could be hurt, and he could be stopped. The whole ordeal would still take some time to get over, but she was getting over it with the help of her new family.

Grady's Pub had been picking up business since the grand re-opening. He was happier than anyone had seen him since before his wife Catie's passing. He had a sense of purpose now, and they both leaned on each other for support, understanding, and love. They helped each other out through those tough days of grief.

Things between Behr and Ellora had grown with each passing day. She still wanted to take things slowly. She wasn't ready yet to take their relationship too far, too fast. After all, this was her first real relationship, and she was in no rush. Naturally, things always seemed to get hot and heavy whenever they were alone together. They were drawn to one another. The pull was more powerful than the strongest magnet. Even when they were separated, it wouldn't last long. An overwhelming need would pull them back to each other. She knew this was the result of Behr witnessing her attack first hand. After he risked his own life without hesitation to protect her, Ellora dropped all guards where he was concerned.

Ellora trusted Behr. She was completely safe with him, both with her life and her heart. She loved him. His intensity and strong feelings toward Ellora no longer set her on edge or scared her. She believed that nothing, or no one, could get to her, so long as she was wrapped securely in his strong, loving arms.

Just like every other day since then, Behr snuck into her second-floor flat located above Grady's Pub. This had become a routine that she looked forward to. She was awakened by the intoxicating aroma of dark, rich, freshly brewed coffee. Ellora was already awake but lay perfectly still, pretending to be asleep, as this was her favorite part of her morning.

Dishes clinked as Behr slid the loaded tray onto her

night stand, then carefully eased his weighty frame into bed beside her. Ellora couldn't help herself; she smiled ear to ear as his large, muscular arm wrapped around her waist. Behr pulled her easily to him, her back to his front. Nuzzling her neck, the love-struck man inhaled her scent deep into his lungs, and sighed contentedly into her hair.

"Mmm, good morning, Behr," the sleepy girl slurred lazily with a deep and raspy voice. The sexy sound roused Behr into action. He rained kisses up and down her neck and on the sensitive spot behind her ear. The tender caresses sent delightful shivers down her spine.

"Mornin', love. Up a little early, are we? I brought your favorite caffeine fix." Obviously tired of talking to her back, he easily lifted and turned her over. Ellora made quick work of covering her mouth. Morning breath was so not sexy. Behr smiled as he grasped her tiny wrists with his large hands, forcefully moving them to her side, ignoring her weak protests.

"Behr, seriously! At least let me go and brush my teeth first!" Her protests fell on deaf ears. The magnificent man continued his delightful assault on her pouty lips, not bothering to heed her warnings, and not seeming to care in the least.

"I love every part of you, Ellora, bad breath and all." He spoke the last words while chuckling against her lips. The rumble of his laughter shook them both. Ellora slapped him a few times playfully at his choice of words. He continued the onslaught on her now pliant lips, and she quickly forgot all about her breath dilemma. All too easily, she got lost in their quiet moment of desire.

Behr's strong mouth pried open her plump lips, delving deep into the kiss. When the first brush of his insistent tongue swept over hers, Ellora let a breathless moan escape. At hearing her reaction and feeling her barely clothed body arching into his, the eager man nearly lost all control. Every time they were together like this, he always pushed her boundaries a little farther, but Behr knew exactly when to slow down and pull away. He knew Ellora, knew how much was too much. Besides, he had a surprise for her today, and they'd never get to it if he didn't drag his arse outta her bed.

Ellora groaned when he pulled away. Oh, God help her, she was falling so hard for this man that it scared her how much she felt for him sometimes. What if he got sick of her... sick of waiting? That thought was always weighing heavily in the back of her mind. But, all she had to do was look into his soulful blue eyes, and all those fleeting thoughts and insecurities would melt away. His affection for her, his love for her, was always gazing right back at her as plain as day.

Behr kissed her neck, cheek, earlobe, and up into her hairline as he spoke to her. "Get. Your. Beautiful. Round arse. Outta this bed. Go 'ave yourself a shower. I 'ave a surprise for you today, love." He kissed her eager lips a few more times before throwing the covers off her and onto the floor, laughing as she groaned her disapproval.

"Get ready, love. I'll meet ya downstairs." Behr laid one more dangerously delicious kiss on her parted lips. Ellora ran her hands up into his thick dark hair, tugging it roughly, while pulling him down on top of her. He never seemed to be close enough to satisfy her. She might not have been ready to go all the way with him yet, but she certainly had uncontrollable and unbridled feelings for Behr that just grew and grew the more time they spent together. He made her want more. She always wanted more when it came to him.

"If you don't release me soon, love, I will never let you out of this bed. I know you're not ready for that yet, so you'd better let me go soon before I forget that I'm a gentleman and change my mind all together." Reaching around, he spanked Ellora's ass hard, unleashing a squeal out of her as he quickly rolled off the bed. Ellora stretched her arms and legs out on the bed, releasing all the kinks and joints from sleep. After a very noisy unladylike yawn, she watched Behr make his way to the door, where he hovered half inside-half outside the door. His eyes roved over her as she lay sprawled out on her messy sheets.

His expression was one she couldn't understand. When their eyes finally met, he smiled so beautifully, it took her breath away. Behr shook his head, in awe of the goddess that lay out before him. "You. Are. Mine," he whispered over to her with pride. Turning on his heels, Behr made his way downstairs. The encounter was quick, and his departure out of the room was just as quick.

Ellora let herself lay in bed a few more peaceful moments, thinking a lot about Behr… About them both. Yes, she was falling in love with him. Easily. She had always been helpless against it. She knew that now.

Hopping out of the bed, the still sleepy girl headed into the bathroom for a long, cold shower to cool down her escalated temperature and desire for the man responsible. She found herself hurrying as she dressed and dried her hair, already anxious to be close to him once again and impatient to find out what his surprise was.

As she made it down the stairs and around to the front of the bar, she could tell she was the topic of everyone's conversation. She was met with silence as soon as she entered. Kristy, Grady's sister-in-law, proved her theory correct as she gave her a big cheesy smile. The motherly woman quickly scooted behind the bar and into the kitchen to grab Ellora some breakfast.

The object of conversation could hear Lachlan express how much 'she'll love it,' in hushed tones to Gavin, while Behr was readying himself to leave. Patrick apparently loved what he was told because his reply was, "Oh, yeah, brother, she will love you forever for this! She will owe you big time."

Curious, she walked in the midst of their conversation with her plate and heavily buttered bagel. She sat on the only available stool, in the center of all the guys. She felt like she had walked onto a *Gone With the Wind* scene, and she was Scarlet O'Hara. "Do I have time to eat?"

Behr strolled over to the owner of his beating heart. "For you… I have all the time in the world. Eat up, love. I'm not going anywhere without you." Ellora blushed scarlet. Oh, this man.

After breakfast, they headed on down Bank Street, and Behr grasped Ellora's hand, lacing their fingers together as he always did. They walked at a slow pace, taking in the unusually warm, sunny morning. Behr led her to the old Armadale building. It was the old hardware store her father used to work at before he'd moved to the States with Ellora's mother. The very same one Giddeon dragged her to, where he had attacked her. A shudder shook her tiny frame at the memory of what took place right here, not so long ago. It was strange; this building held such fond memories of Ellora and Behr's first date, and the heart-stopping story of her parents' love-at-first-sight encounter in this very same location. But, it was also the site of terrible encounters and nightmarish close calls.

The different feelings and thoughts were confusing for her. But, the good seemed to outweigh the bad, because every time she stood outside this building, she thought of her parents and how much she loved and missed them. Hope swelled inside her chest as they stepped closer. She stood in front of the abandoned building and stared at the bright yellow sign that read 'FOR LEASE'. Ellora's head whipped around, and she glanced up at Behr. A knowing smile was already in place as he nodded at her. Ellora couldn't help but answer his silent gesture with a smile of her own.

"I think it's about time for you to get your career started, love. Grady's place is fixed up n' runnin' successfully because of you. Now, it's time for Ellora Belle Sutherland to start living her life. You could start your own contractor's business 'ere." He waved his hand at yet another sad looking building that begged for some TLC—one that called out to her to be restored. "The lease is reasonable, and best of all, it's centrally located in town."

Behr ran his hand down her cheek, skimming it gently with his fingertips, and cupped her chin. Turning her head around and up to meet his eyes, he told her, "You can do this, love. I know ya can. I will be 'ere by your side every step of the way. You deserve all the happiness this world has to offer. Your father and mother would want this for you, as well, so I will do whatever it takes to make sure it happens."

Behr lifted one eyebrow and smirked when he caught Ellora's tell-tale, 'I'm about to cry' chin tremble. "Let's just say I'm acting on their behalf."

Tears filled her eyes and threatened to spill over at the

very mention of her loving parents. Her chest ached as she was consumed by the hollowness and sorrow that resided inside her broken heart. She wished, like always, that they could be here with her. But, now, she had a new wish to add to it. She wished her dad could've met Behr. He would've liked him a great deal. "You're right, Behr. This is exactly what my parents would've wanted for me."

The thoughtful man kissed the tip of her nose and nibbled her quivering chin before breaking their eye contact. He looked back over to the abandoned warehouse, rubbing his forefinger and thumb along his stubbled chin, deep in thought.

"I think we might be able to strike up a bargain with the Leaser in much the same way you did with Grady. Lower the lease amount, and in exchange, we could fix up all the property damage on our own, saving them the hassle and cost."

This building had suffered a lot of damage. Giddeon broke the side door in order to carry out his plan to forcefully bring Ellora back to Dalton. The bay windows were completely busted out. Shattered glass littered all over the floor on the inside. The walls and sheet rock were cracked in some areas and suffered huge holes in others, due to their fight. Add to that decades of abandonment and neglect. This. Place. Was. Trashed.

Her heart raced in panic at the thought of someone else possibly getting their hands on this property. It was, after all, an amazing deal. What if they took over and tore it all down to the ground to rebuild? Starting over from scratch *would* be the easiest thing to do. But, this was her father's hardware store... and his father's before him. He met her mother here. He fell in love with her right inside this very building.

Even in its depressing, ominous state, she could still feel the loving presence of her parents all around her. Ellora closed her eyes and let the warm sun wrap itself around her like a mother's embrace. She could sense them and all the years of good memories that came with this building. It was now the only possession Ellora could get her hands on that was directly connected to her parents. She couldn't let anyone else have it. She wouldn't even entertain the thought. That warehouse belonged to her, belonged in her family line alone.

In some odd way, the run-down building looked as though it cried out for someone to show mercy and compassion for its sad state. Just like Ellora, it needed a lot of hard work and love to get it back to the way it used to be. Fixing it up might be therapeutic. Ellora would work on the building... and in a way, the building would work on her. It wouldn't be easy, but it was worth every effort.

Behr was right; Grady's place was finished. It was finally time for her to stop hiding and start living her life the way she wanted. She could do this. Ellora looked up at Behr as excitement grew steadily inside of her. He tilted his head to the side and grinned a lopsided grin, waiting for her answer. She brought herself up on her tiptoes, so she could reach his lips, and laid a kiss that could melt ice. Behr's eyebrows flew up in surprise.

"Yes! This building's been in my family for years. It's mine. Always has been. Let's make the call. I want to get started immediately."

Behr wrapped his arms around her waist, lifting her up and twirling her around in circles. She giggled as a surge of excited anticipation and nervousness pulsed through her veins at the thought of actually being a business owner. Ellora kissed Behr while still in his arms, and savored the warmth of his lips. His strong, full lips moved against hers with the perfect amount of pressure. It had her soaring higher and higher into a pleasure she had yet to understand.

Behr captured her bottom lip with his teeth and pulled, letting out a rough throaty laugh when Ellora squeaked out her surprise. Landing one more peck on the tip of her nose, Behr finally decided to set her back down on solid ground. Pulling his cell out of his pocket, Ellora watched as his strong hands balanced the delicate device, his large fingers skillfully punching in the numbers. He pressed it to his ear and waited.

"Yes. Hello, Miss, I'm calling about a property you have listed for lease. May I have a moment to speak with the agent in charge, please? Aye, I can hold." Behr's eyes shifted to focus back on Ellora.

"There's no better time than here and now. Your future has been here waiting for you all along, Ellora. Grab it with both hands, love. Hang on for the ride...."

The ecstatic girl in his arms nodded in agreement. She squeezed him in tighter, finishing his sentence. "...And never let go."

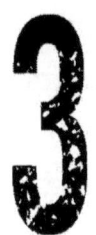

iddeon didn't know how Dominick convinced the Scottish authorities, or the angry townsfolk, to let him go, but they were definitely not happy about it. Their flight back to Syracuse was long and exhausting. Detective Antonelli replaced his cuffs with an expensive, state of the art ankle bracelet with a GPS tracking device directly connected to his cell phone. Dominick was just one click away from knowing his exact whereabouts. Yes. There is an app for that.

Their flight was relatively quiet, as they were both engulfed in their own thoughts. A lot had happened in a short period of time. Dominick informed him right off the bat that he would be staying with him that night. He didn't want Giddeon out of his sight for one minute. He didn't blame him, either. This didn't bother Giddeon in the slightest; hardly anything did anymore. Plus, it was a way better set up than prison.

Giddeon was numbly going through all the motions, still in shock over the events that had unfolded.

When they arrived, Dominick steered them straight to his apartment to catch up on some much need rest, unpack, and unwind, which was fine with him. He wasn't sure yet where they would start on their mutual quest to take down Dalton. After all, they couldn't just march through his high-rise office, accusing him of disappearances and multiple homicides... or, at the very least, of being the mastermind behind all of it. They needed evidence to back it up, and trustworthy people to follow through with the prosecution. The second would be harder to find. Dalton had very powerful friends in very high places.

He was smarter than that, anyway. Giddeon would bet that Dalton already knew they were back in town. He would definitely be looking over his shoulder for the remainder of the time he was in the city.

Giddeon realized, too late, that he had absolutely zilch with him. No clothes. No toothbrush. No possessions of any kind. And he desperately needed a shower. Swallowing his dwindling pride, he walked into the living room. Dominick lounged all the way back in his dark, beat up, leather recliner, aimlessly flipping through the TV channels. "Hey, Detective, you got any clothes I can bum off you until I collect all my shit from my place?"

"Yeah. Sure." Dominick let out an exhausted breath as he hauled himself up out of the comfortable chair. "No problem." He followed him down the short narrow hallway a few steps behind, to the last room on the right. Giddeon hung back, not wanting to invade his personal space. He leaned his worn out body on the threshold of the creaky door.

Dominick pulled out a couple pairs of graphic t-shirts, a pair of dark faded jeans, and a grey pair of sweatpants. He tossed them in his direction. "You're going to have to free ball it until we go get your stuff, because there is no way in hell you're wearing my fucking boxers."

Ha. What a smart ass, Giddeon thought, smirking as he passed by him. "What? Are you telling me we're not going to be BFFs? That hurts my feelings, Detective," Giddeon gave back, heavy on the sarcasm.

Dominick shook his head in defeat, laughing lightly. "Shut up, asshole, and stop calling me Detective in my own house. It's getting weird."

Dominick flung his hand out, motioning toward a smaller door adjacent to his bedroom door. "The bathroom is through there, and for the love of God… use your own bar of soap. Fresh bars are in the cabinet under the sink."

"Thanks, boss." Giddeon nodded, appreciating the fresh digs. He walked into the small bathroom and paused halfway in, turning around as a thought popped into his head. But, he was interrupted before he even got the chance to ask.

"Bracelet's waterproof," Dominick shouted over his shoulder without looking back, as he headed back over to his waiting chair.

Six-thirty rolled around, and Dominick finally dragged himself out of the chair and into the kitchen.

Groggily, he filled a well-worn pot with water and placed it on his older model stove. Giddeon walked into the kitchen with his hair still dripping from his heavenly hot shower. He hadn't had one that relaxing in a while. "Whatcha makin' for dinner, Dad?" he asked with a condescending voice, trying his best to get under his skin.

Dominick answered him quickly, not at all phased by his personality. "Ramen Noodles."

Giddeon pumped his fist in the air enthusiastically. "Yes. We're eating like kings tonight. Woohoo! All right!" He smirked when the detective glanced over at him, and he knew what he was thinking, too. 'God. What. A. Prick.'

Instead, he chuckled dryly, adding, "You play your cards right, and we'll eat like this every night." Giddeon pulled out a chair and plopped down heavily at the table in the eat-in kitchen. He was surprised that he couldn't get a rise out of Dominick. He seemed willing to play along.

Scooping up two big spoonfuls, he dumped them into big soup bowls. Dominick slid Giddeon's across the table at him, sagged down into his own chair, and dug in. They wasted no time shoveling the noodles into their mouths hungrily. Dominick eyed him the whole time. Giddeon could see he wanted to ask him some questions. *Cops.*

"What's on your mind, Dom? Spit it out."

Taking one more big bite, he gulped hard and answered. "I was just wondering how you came into contact with Dalton? How did you meet him?"

Still eating, Giddeon snorted at that question. He kicked his leg up onto the chair he was sitting in, and draped his arm over his knee. Screw manners—this was how he always ate. Why stop now? "Online dating. No, wait... It was an ad in the personals."

Dominick dropped his spoon down into his empty bowl, making a clanking sound, and just glared at him. His frustration with him finally showed in the ticking of his jaw.

"All right, all right, I'm just fucking with you. Keep your panties on." Giddeon slurped down a spoonful of soggy noodles as he thought back to the very first encounter. He started the story even with his mouth full.

"Well, after my..." Nope. His brain put a halt to his big mouth before he revealed more. Refusing to talk about his parents, he skipped ahead. "I hated my foster parents. They were dicks. So, I used to sneak out of the house every chance I got and would wander around downtown. There was this one skater shop and tattoo joint I liked to hang out at, to people watch. Or pick fights. Mostly, pick fights. Well, there was this high class rich man's club a few buildings down. This thick-necked, juice using asshole stood out front. I guess he was supposed to be a bouncer. I couldn't stand looking at his fat face anymore, so I messed with him non-stop, trying to find that one button, that one button everyone has that prevents them from snapping, and press it. It didn't take me long at all to find his and push."

Dominick raised one eyebrow at the man sitting

across from him, prompting him to go on. He was obviously curious as to what it was.

"I asked him if his girlfriend had to use a magnifying glass to find his dick. His face turned purple, and he roared at me… like, actually roared out like a lion. I apologized and said, 'My bad, bro. I meant your boyfriend." I told him he better quit the 'roids before his micro-penis regressed into a vagina, and he wouldn't be able to please his boyfriend anymore."

Dominick threw his head back and bellowed out a long throaty laugh. He hadn't laughed in a long time. His lungs hurt from the force of it, the sound echoing off the walls in the cramped kitchen. Giddeon laughed right along with him. "Anyone ever tell you that you have a serious anger problem?"

His inked arms flew out to his sides. "That I do, Detective," he agreed, still laughing. "Well, he charged me like a raging bull. I swear I saw smoke coming out of his eyes and ears. He lunged at me, slow and clumsy. I easily dodged out of his way and kicked my foot out, tripping him and shouting 'Timber' as he went down. He fell hard on the paved walkway. I jumped on top of him, pounding the piss out of him. Come to find out, that club… and that meathead, belonged to Dalton."

Pausing the story, Giddeon finished up his poor man's meal, grabbed the bowl, and walked into the kitchen. He dumped the bowl into the sink, hopped up onto the counter top, and continued. "I was a kid full of incredible anger with no way of unleashing it all. I couldn't control it, and I definitely couldn't stop once I'd started."

Giddeon hesitated, running his marked-up hands through his damp hair. "Hell, I still can't. That wasn't the first time I picked a fight for no reason, but it *was* the one that changed everything. As I rained punches down on his bloodied face, a noise pulled me out of my destructive haze. I was distracted by the loud clicking noise of a Zippo lighter. Dalton was leaning up against the club doors, a cigar firmly in hand. He just watched as I demolished his goon. His smile was dripping with self-righteous arrogance, and it stopped me dead in my tracks. I eased up off the meathead and stood up to face him. Not sure what would happen next, I readied myself for either another fight, or to run the hell outta there."

Giddeon aimlessly rearranged the items lined up on Dominick's countertop for another minute. He did this until Dominick drew his attention back by asking, "What did he do with you?"

He looked over at him, still sitting at the table. "I remember thinking that this yuppie asshole was going to call the cops for sure. But, instead, he assured me that he never involved the police in his affairs. He looked down at his goon with disgust, which shocked me, and then regarded me, apparently impressed with what I'd done.

"After instructing one of his men to drag the goon off

the street, he bargained with me instead. He pledged to forget all about this incident, but only if I came to work for him in his new building. I'd start out at the bottom, of course... A janitor. I don't know if that was like a metaphor for 'clean up your act' or whatever. But, he was going to pay me well, so I thought what the hell. I moved up the ranks quickly." Giddeon shrugged as he ended the story right there.

Dominick leaned far back in his chair, balancing on the two back legs and drumming his fingers on the table top. Giddeon could tell the direction the detective's thoughts were taking him by the look on his face.

"When was the first incident he had you threaten or hurt someone? And who was it?"

And there it was. A burning churned heavily in the pit of Giddeon's stomach and grew outward. He pinched the bridge of his nose as anger, guilt, and regret seemed to cloud over his vision. He tried hard to focus on his end goal... Getting his hands on Dalton... Find and kill the man responsible for butchering his parents. When Dominick got up from the chair, Giddeon quickly jumped off the counter.

He paced back and forth in the cramped space, trying without success to relieve his pent up aggression and extra energy. Without some sort of an outlet, it always took him a while to get a hold of himself. That familiar need deep inside him grew. He shook with the effort it took to restrain himself from smashing everything around him, and maiming the first person he could get his hands on. Air whooshed in and out of his lungs in short, shallow breaths.

"Not now, Detective... Not tonight. I... just. Can't." Unconsciously, he cracked his knuckles as he thought about the vile, horrendous things Dalton had him do in those early years. Giddeon despised himself. Cold sweat broke out on his forehead as the dangerously familiar need itched and clawed its way out of him, prickling all across his skin. Begging him to hurt someone... to hurt himself. Giddeon's tremors grew more violent. He knew he had to try to control *this* while staying here.

Dominick casually strode back into the kitchen. Too close to Giddeon. "Stay away from me." His voice was several octaves lower, anger and frustration altering the sound. "I just... need a minute. Give me a minute to get myself right." Through the thrumming in his ears, he was aware of Dominick's heavy footsteps as he walked by him. Too close. Giddeon turned his back, unable to face him in this state. Grabbing the edge of the countertop, the deeply disturbed man gripped them with a force that whitened his knuckles under the punishing pressure.

Dominick opened the fridge, and a few seconds later, a can of beer skidded across the Formica surface toward him. "I'll give you a few days to settle in. Then, we are having this conversation. You got that?"

Struggling with his slipping control, he couldn't answer. He couldn't even turn around to look at him. He was ready to lose it at any moment. He acknowledged him by one simple nod. Dominick pointed at him with the beer can still in his hand. "We'll stop by your place tomorrow to pick up your shit, a'right?"

He guzzled his beer then tossed the empty can under the sink. "I've had enough of this shit for one day. I'm racking out. Don't try to run or something stupid like that. You'll just set off the alarm, and it's annoying as hell. So don't do it or all bets are off." The detective must've believed Giddeon wouldn't run, because his statement was made without any passionate threats and in passing.

Giddeon finally turned, yelling out after him as he walked down the hall, "I'm not going anywhere, not until my business is finally finished.

They headed over to Giddeon's apartment building first thing the next morning, to pick up some of his stuff. Giddeon shuffled down the cement steps to his basement apartment. He always chose places on or around ground level. There had to be several exit points available… just in case. It had become an obsessive necessity after the death of his parents. He glanced down as he pulled out the key from his borrowed pants pocket.

With the correct key in hand, Giddeon glanced up, noticing for the first time that the front door was opened a crack. The wooden frame by the lock had been damaged. "FUCK!" he whisper-shouted, thinking how Karma's a bitch and was catching up to him fast after the terrible things he'd done to others. Innocent people like Ellora. Dominick stepped forward and unholstered his gun.

He scolded Giddeon through a strained whispered voice that Dominick tried hard to keep low. "Keep your voice down. We don't know if someone is still in there. Now, get behind me so I can clear the apartment first."

"Give me back my dagger, Detective. I don't know what's in there. I'm not going in unprotected." Dominick gave him an apprehensive 'no way in hell' look.

"Listen, I'm not going to use it on anyone, okay. I just... *need* it back. It has significant value to me. I won't hurt anyone until I find Dalton, all right?"

Dominick shot him a hard glare as he reached into his side cargo pocket. He handed over his dagger, but at the last minute, he hesitated and pulled back. "You're not going to kill him, either. I want the satisfaction of watching him slowly rot in prison. Understand?"

Yeah right, Giddeon thought to himself. "Sure, Detective. I won't kill him." He raised both hands in a peaceful gesture, mimicking a scout's honor, trying hard to placate him. "I already told you... I have an agenda. I help you, you help me, right? Well, I'll really need your help when this is all over. Okay?"

Dominick offered up a half-crooked grin and nodded

in response, handing over the dagger. Immediately, a calm relief settled over Giddeon. He had just been thrown his life line. This piece was his only link to a violent past. It was a reminder of what he had to do. What he *needed* to do.

Giddeon kicked his door noisily. It bounced off the wall, leaving a big door knob sized dent. Ignoring Dominick's order to stand behind him, Giddeon plowed right through, marching right in. No fear. Never any fear.

Dominick rushed in behind him, cursing the whole way because of Giddeon's careless stunt. "Stupid asshole. Why don't you just announce to the world that we're coming in?"

The agitated man stood in what used to be his front room. Half empty, wiped clean, abandoned. "Shit! He's erasing me," Giddeon shouted. Anger bubbled up inside him at the realization. He turned and ran down the hallway to the last room, bursting through his bedroom door. He was taken aback, as there was nothing much left behind. What little remained was trashed or broken. No furniture was left behind. Shouting out in frustration, he unleashed his growing fury on the wall closest to him. His fists connected in a flurry, leaving big gaping holes in the sheetrock.

After enough time passed, Giddeon was able to get himself back under control and calm down. He started searching through the rubble left in his closet. He was able to find a couple pairs of pants, a shirt, and a few pairs of boxers—dirty, but intact. Shoving his belongings in a plastic grocery bag he found close by, he headed back out to the living room to join Dominick. He found him kneeling on the ground, where his end table used to be, just staring at something.

Giddeon walked up behind him, glancing over his shoulder. "Looks like I'm going to be rooming with you for a little while longer."

Dominick held up one hand with an object dangling from it. "Hey, man, I found these. They're in pretty good shape… You want 'em?" He held up faded, black wooden beads and passed them over.

Giddeon sank to his knees and closed his eyes, thankful that they hadn't been ruined. "Yes. I do." Carefully taking them from the detective's hands, he looked over them like they were the most precious treasure ever found.

"These were my mother's." He caressed the beautifully carved beads fondly in the palm of his hand. "She carried these with her everywhere. She went to mass every Wednesday and Sunday. This is the only thing I have left that belonged to her." The last sentence made it past his lips in a hushed whisper. He placed a gentle kiss on the precious heirloom, rose to his feet, and looked over to Dominick, who had wandered into the kitchen.

A renewed sense of vengeance helped to once again clear his vision. "All right. Let's get the hell outta here." Giving one more loving kiss on his mother's rosary, Giddeon placed it around his neck and walked out of his past and into a more purposeful future. He had to keep focused. He would get his revenge… or die trying.

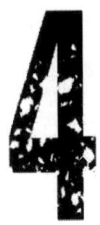

"So, what's up, Dom? What're we doing? What's the plan?" The car ride had been a silent one after leaving Giddeon's place. Curiosity got the better of him, which opened him up a little bit. They were headed inside Saint Joseph's Hospital. The last time he was in there, he was following Dalton's orders to shadow the detective and report back to him. His thoughts about what went down in the recent past, and how much things had changed, must've slowed his pace.

He jogged to get in step with Dominick as he passed through the hospital's double doors. "I've got a couple questions to ask my girl. She helped me out a lot when I was trying to locate Ellora." Giddeon knew a few of the nurses caught him the night he snuck into Ellora's room as she recovered from his attack. A wave of guilt crashed over him as visions of her terrified expression drifted into his head. He would've finished her off right there, too, had it not been for all the chaos happening right outside her room.

There were just too many people around. He wouldn't have been able to enjoy himself in the process. Thinking back on it now, he was glad she lived. There were brief moments in Portree where he empathized with Ellora, knowing full well what was waiting for her back in Syracuse, for what he was planning to put her through... for what he'd already done to her.

Because of his blind loyalty for Dalton, he'd killed her parents. He ripped them out of her life, just as someone ripped his parents out of his life. She didn't deserve it, either. She didn't deserve any of it.

Giddeon shrunk in on himself as self-loathing took over. He was the biggest piece of shit garbage that ever walked the earth. Giddeon literally turned into the thing he hated most, the very monsters he was hunting down. Shaking off his self-hatred, he quickened his pace. What's done was done. Knowing what he did now, Giddeon would've changed things if he could. But, like always, he was too late.

"This should be interesting. I wonder what they'll think of our partnership? Good and evil unite forces to defeat a common enemy... Stay tuned."

Giddeon smirked as Dominick looked back with a humorless sideways glance. "What, partner? Sick of me already?"

Dominick just shook his head, mumbling, "I love you about as much as a hemorrhoid on a hot day!"

Giddeon nodded, rubbing his chin. "That much, huh? Wow, that's a step up, Detective. I'm flattered."

They walked up to the registration desk. Dominick

approached a young lady as Giddeon turned, taking in his surroundings. The waiting room was packed with a diverse group of anxious patients—some sick, some bleeding, and others laid out on stretchers. A few more rolled in on wheelchairs. The smell of blood and sickness wafted around the room, while the powerful odor of bleach competed to mask the offending odors. He had always loved the sounds, smells, and general atmosphere inside hospitals. Giddeon glanced over his shoulder at Dominick, whose back faced him, blocking his view of the woman behind the counter.

After a while, it sounded like she was giving him a hard time. "Where is Vicky? Isn't she supposed to be working today? I need you to tell me where I can find her. It's extremely important." His questions poured out of his mouth in rapid succession. "Listen, Sir… Vicky is not here, nor will she be anytime soon. So, how can I help you?"

Her attitude had Giddeon snapping his head back. He had to tamp down the stirring beast within before he approached her. Stalking up alongside his oddly matched partner, Giddeon readied himself to rip the person a new one. Instead, he was met by the most stunning creature he had ever laid his eyes on, with the cutest scowl pointed right at him, which threw him completely off guard.

The curious man halted his movements abruptly. Inconveniently, his tongue was completely tied. This was all new to him. He always had a smart mouth ready and waiting to talk shit… until right then. Giddeon slowly stepped closer to the desk, needing to get closer to her.

This woman's eyes were very unique—a brilliant, tropical, ocean blue with a darker blue ring around the irises. They drew him in, and he was now staring powerlessly at her. She had sharp cheek bones that jutted out perfectly, like a carved sculpture of a goddess come to life. She was definitely rocking an ethereal, otherworldly look. Her irresistibly full, soft looking lips were shaped like Cupid's bow. And that hair... golden, shimmering and silky. The gleaming strands must have been spun from pure gold. She wore it in a high pony tail, hanging long and curling at the ends.

Giddeon's fingers itched to pull out the elastic and watch as her hair cascaded down around her shoulders, as he imagined it would probably do. A gravel-rough voice brought the man down and out of the clouds that he was hovering in, when Dominick loudly coughed, clearing his throat. He jabbed him hard with his elbow, snapping the day-dreamer out of his momentary haze.

Ummm... okay. This man is straight up staring at me. Scratch that. He looks as though he's trying to use mind control on me, Eva thought to herself. Geez, if looks could kill, she'd be six feet under. The way his stone-faced, black eyes bore into her, looked like he could crush her skull with the power of his mind alone. Scary stuff.

"Um, excuse me… What are you staring at?" The dark stranger didn't answer back, just stared. Oddly enough, his expression seemed to transform the longer he stared. Eva's cheeks flushed as his eyes roved over her, slow and deliberate, from the top of her head to the soles of her feet and back again. The cryptic man made no attempt to hide his obvious study.

How would she describe this man…? Dark. Definitely handsome in the dangerous bad-boy kinda way, but disturbing at the same time. His eyes, at first glance, looked midnight black, but obviously were a very dark brown. They were large and alarming, unsettling to her at first. They were lined with equally dark brows and lashes to match. His floppy, just-out-of-bed mess of black hair added to his sinister appearance.

He had a lot of elaborate tattoos peeking out of the collar and sleeves of his t-shirt, weaving down both arms into full sleeves. Talons seemed to claw their way up his neck, accentuating a large, jagged scar that ran horizontally across his neck. As she continued her assessment of his appearance, she noticed that he had another jagged scar running through his eyebrow, but it was well hidden.

This man looked like he'd battled his way out of hell… and prevailed. If she looked past all those things, his lean toned physique and facial bone structure were flawless. After a minute of their mutual staring contest, Eva looked at the man next to him... and shrugged. His closely cropped cut and aviator sunglasses screamed cop. "What's this guy's problem, huh?" The cop looking guy cleared his throat and nudged the dark man with his elbow. Eva crossed her arms over her chest and waited as he blinked several times. When she was sure he was mentally all there, she placed her hands on her hips, asking, yet again, "What's your problem? What are you looking at?"

The man's legs forged a path toward the girl, his eyes narrowing their attention on her. He lifted the corner of his lip in a lopsided grin which looked both sinister and cocky.

Great. He's playing with me and obviously thinks it's amusing, she grumbled to herself.

"An angel."

His voice did funny things in the pit of her stomach. It was both a soft whisper and a deep raspy growl. She didn't like it... *Because* she liked it.

"Don't call me that." Eva's voice came out harsher than she wanted it to sound. She watched him carefully as his eyes slowly dragged their way down to her name tag that rested just above her left breast. He raised a challenging brow. "Name tag says Ev-*Angel*-ina." He dragged out the syllables, purposefully separating "angel" just to make his point.

Eva rolled her eyes, heavy on the attitude. "Only my grandparents call me that. Since you aren't... call me Eva... P L E A S E." She forced out the please, her tone dripping with annoyance.

The cop, obviously tired of their banter back and forth, shook his head in agitation. "Listen, I need to ask her some questions. She was helping me with a case not too long ago."

Eva pointed an accusing finger at him. "Oh, so you're the one she risked her life helping, huh? Yeah. She spoke about you before she slipped into a coma. Nice job, dude."

The cop's face snapped up in surprise, reddening at this news. "Did... did you just say she's in a coma?" Eva took her hand off her hip and crossed them again, nodding slowly.

Dominick turned his head, giving his dark partner an eerily icy glare. The dark man lifted his hands and laughed at him, not fazed by the look at all. "Whoa, don't look at me like that, Detective... Wasn't me. Didn't do it."

Eva couldn't help but wonder why he would think the man he came in with would have anything to do with it. Yup. He was definitely a dangerous man, all right. One she better stay away from. An arctic chill crawled up her spine, leaving goosebumps to follow, as she watched him. And it wasn't from fear.

Yes. Eva was one of those women who were helplessly and instantly drawn to bad boys. But, this man... was different somehow. He wasn't faking it like most guys did. There was something sinister hidden deep down inside of him. God help her, she was immediately attracted to him.

Both men now stood by, waiting for her to say something, showing their growing annoyance with her lack of cooperation. The dark one blew out an exaggerated breath and leaned over the small desk. Eva wasn't sure how he did it, but his expression flickered along with the dull lighting overhead. A shadow passed over him, morphing his previously blatant flirtation to a bone-chilling, cold, and murderous glare. Charles Manson himself would've been impressed with it. His disdainful malice and offensive stance as he towered over her with clenched fists implied his attempt to intimidate her.

Nope! You don't scare me, my dark stallion. Think again, Eva thought to herself. Lifting up the counter partition, she passed through and marched directly into his space, undeterred by his menacing presence. Cocking her head to the side, Eva defiantly glowered right back at him.

The dark stranger must be used to scaring men and women alike, because he appeared shocked for a fleeting moment at her in-your-face challenge. Determination grew inside of him as he bent down over her, pointing a finger in her chest. With a harsh whisper, he threatened, "Where. Is. The. Girl? If you don't tell me quickly, I will go out of my way to make sure you regret that decision."

"Oooooh, really?" Eva laughed long and hard. Who did this guy think he was? "Honey, please. I work the addiction wing and head up the anger management support group." Straightening her spine with outrage, she stood up on tiptoes and jabbed her finger in his chest, mimicking him. The moment her hand touched him, the man hissed through tightly clenched teeth. At the point of contact, his dark expression was shaken clean like an etch-a-sketch. A ghost of a smile threatened to appear.

"I have seen and heard more despicably horrific nightmares than you could ever possibly imagine up in that tiny, useless brain of yours. If you're trying to scare me, you'd better think again. Or try harder at it. Either way, I. Am. Not. Scared. Of. You."

Eva glanced over at his stunned partner. "What's with this guy? Does he always act like this?" Not knowing what else to do in this unexpected altercation, Dominick eyed the pair and nodded exasperatedly. "Oh, okay. That explains everything... You're just an incredible dickhead. Well, that's too bad. There's no cure for that." The feisty girl lifted her head in defiance, daring him to say something else.

Both men's eyes widened at hearing the foul, crass language coming from the beautiful, petite girl. The cop looked her over, then his eyes drifted to his dark partner and took in his surprise. Giddeon wasn't the sort of man who became tongue-tied easily, and Dominick was entertained by his dumbstruck appearance. Dominick belted out a laugh that captured the attention of the rest of the waiting room, who all whipped their heads around in their direction. "I love this girl. She's not afraid of you and won't take any of your shit, Giddeon."

Unable to help herself, Eva laughed right along with him, loving the sound of his infectious cackling. "Giddeon, huh?" Eva tested out the name over and over inside her head and decided that she liked the way it rolled off her tongue. He nodded once, relaxing his stance a few fractions as the tension eased in the small space around them.

Eva studied Giddeon once more and bit her lip. "The mighty destroyer… Well, that name definitely suits you." Eva was big into name meanings. His was biblical and definitely fit his demeanor. Giddeon kept on nodding and smirked at her ruthlessly.

"Oh, you have no idea how close you've hit the mark, Angel." He paused to allow his onyx eyes to rove over her curvaceous figure one more time before switching tactics. Softening his voice as best he could, Giddeon relaxed his stance. "Is there any way we can see that girl today? Talk to her?"

Eva shook her head. "You can't talk to someone if they can't talk." She pulled a card out of her pocket. "Here's my card with all the appropriate numbers to reach me. You can call every day at those hours listed on the back. Call with questions, concerns, or updates. I will let you know when she wakes, okay."

Eva stretched her arm over, handing the cop the card. He was obviously the one in charge, but Giddeon snatched it out of her hand. Unease crept up inside her as she watched the dark man intimately stroke the proffered card lovingly with his fingers. The attention he gave the item made her stomach churn. He outlined all the words and numbers before putting it in his back pocket.

The cop walked closer to her, eyeing Giddeon suspiciously before bringing his eyes back to her. "Thank you, Eva. I will check on her daily. Umm... What happened to her? Vicky, I mean?" His concern had her retracting her claws she previously unleashed, softening up a fraction.

"Vicky was attacked in her car, outside the hospital parking lot. She was beaten pretty badly. By the time help arrived, she was unconscious and non-responsive. She slipped into a coma soon after." Eva looked directly in the cop's eyes and let him have it. "It was the night she went out to meet you. The police on scene said it was a robbery. Her canvas bag was missing, as well as several other items from her car.

Dominick's eyes narrowed into slits, then widened as something dawned on him. He let out a deep sorrowful sigh, squeezing his eyes shut tightly.

Eva continued. "Vicky had told me that night that she was meeting up with a detective for dinner, to give information on a missing girl that had stayed here." Eva could tell right then and there that this was the very same detective. The sorrowful guilt displayed on his face made that quite clear.

"I never meant for her to get hurt. Thank you again, Eva. We'll stop by again later to check up on her. I'm

Detective Dominick Antonelli, by the way."

They finally shook hands, and he briefly laid a grief-stricken hand on her shoulder, before turning on his heel and walking out the door. "Goodbye, Detective."

Giddeon had a fleeting bout of jealous possessiveness the moment the detective touched her, envious that he hadn't. *Huh, boys,* she thought.

"Oh, and Angel..."

Eva risked a glance over at Giddeon, annoyed that he still insisted on calling her that. "What is it?"

His eyes warmed over a fraction, almost materializing as dark chocolate pools. "I'm sorry about your friend." Eva nodded her reply as he followed Dominick out the doors.

Giddeon was on her mind the rest of the day. Something about his eyes called out to her. They were both forlorn and malicious. Her confused feelings warred within her. On the one hand, Eva hoped she'd never encounter them again. On the other, she prayed she would get the chance to once again feel them as they bore deep into hers.

One thing was certain; she couldn't wait to see him again. And that is why she had to stay away from that man. Giddeon was trouble.

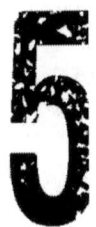

"**P**lease, God. Please take me, too. Don't leave me here... Don't leave me all alone. I want to be with my mommy and daddy... I'm scared." The boy wasn't sure how long it'd been. He'd been lying there beside his parents for a long time, unwilling to leave their side and not knowing what else to do.

The sun had risen high in the sky when it happened, and like a broken movie stuck on pause, there he stood. Too scared to move, daylight soon disappeared, leaving him frozen and petrified in the growing darkness... just as his parents were. Shock had kept him motionless all night, unable to process the horror he'd witnessed.

The sun had risen hours ago, bringing the lost boy out of his stupor. The warm glow of the summer rays shone through the window and onto his frozen face, awakening him out of one nightmare and throwing him into a new kind of hell. The heat coming in signaled that it was around lunch time. When his young consciousness switched back on, he was finally able to move. He'd dropped down beside them, willing his stiffened limbs to move, and reached out a trembling hand to shake them softly. "Mommy, wake up. They're gone now."

Desperately needing the comfort, the little boy struggled to get her unmoving form to hug him back. But, her arm wouldn't budge. She was unnaturally hard, like the sitting stone in the backyard... and unnaturally cold. Not even his favorite Ironman blankie would warm her. His little arms draped over her, shivering as he nestled in closer to the unfeeling object, trying his best to cover her.

She smelled bad. The putrid stench drifted with the breeze across his face. The overwhelming power of the decaying flesh made his eyes and nose sting as painful tears pricked his dry eyes. But he didn't care, nuzzling into his mother's ungiving arms with the eagerness of a desperate child. He'd have done anything to get them to wake up, to come back to him... to hold him and tell him everything was going to be okay. That he was safe.

He tried to pull her resisting body tighter. "Why won't she hug me back?" His fear grew as time ticked by, sitting all alone in this terrifyingly quiet house. Hot tears rolled down his paling cheeks. "I want to be where you are. I want to be in heaven with you, Mommy and Daddy." The little boy shivered against the frigid body beside him. "I don't want to be here all alone."

He jumped when he heard thunderous pounding, banging at the front door. He curled up in a tight ball against his mommy's cold hard side, trying frantically to hide himself. The shivering little boy held his breath, willing himself to hold still, but his terrified body couldn't stop shaking. The blanket vibrated with each violent tremor.

"The monsters are back to hurt me, too." His voice cracked as he whispered to the iron figure lying next to him. He pulled his blankie up over his head, too afraid to see who was coming. Footsteps echoed through the house as the strangers made their way into the room adjacent to the terrified boy. He sucked in stale air and held his breath, too frightened that he'd make a sound. The footsteps stomped louder as they drew closer... coming straight toward the panicked boy.

Giddeon clutched the dagger that still lay wrapped in his hands, close to his chest. The closer they approached, the tighter he clenched the dagger. His fingers tingled with numbness from the lack of movement. His erratic heart was thumping much too fast. His chest ached from the punishment. He was distracted by the hammering of his overworked heart as it thudded loud in his ears. Time stood still as the young boy lay motionless, waiting for something to happen. After a while, he realized that he couldn't hear their footsteps anymore. It had become really quiet.

Still unsure, he laid perfectly still. Are they gone? He wondered. His little ears rang as he strained them to hear something... to hear anything at all. The silence was deafening. He couldn't wait any longer, his curiosity getting the better of him. Just one little peak. He had to know if the monsters were gone.

Bit by bit, he lifted the blankie...

It was ripped away from the alarmed boy. Too terrified

to look, he pinched his eyes shut and screamed at the top of his lungs. And didn't stop.

Giddeon woke to the sound of his own screams.

"Fuck!" He jerked upright, twisting in the blankets of his sweat dampened bed. His sheets were soaked through and sticking to his heated skin. Beads of sweat dripped down his temple, and he struggled to get a grip on his lingering grief, disoriented by the ringing in his ears. Hyperventilating, Giddeon pulled in ragged, painful breaths.

He could still feel their cold bodies up against his... could still smell the powerful memory of their long dead stench, lingering in his nose. Suffocating from his accelerated heartrate, Giddeon tried to control and steady his panicked breathing, desperate to get the nightmarish images out of his head. Tears that hadn't been shed in over a decade were streaming down his ashen face.

The crippling ache in his chest, the ache reserved for the memory of his parents, was ripped wide open after reliving the hellish nightmare. The loss, the loneliness, and the overwhelming guilt left him painfully raw and hollow inside. He couldn't handle that kind of sorrow and torment. It was all too much for him. Too many excruciating emotions clawed at him all at once, and he just couldn't handle it. Giddeon was accustomed to feeling nothing at all. Living a life numb and void was better than living with the gut-wrenching ache that ripped him apart from the inside out every time he caught a glimpse of that sickening nightmare. Some things were better left forgotten.

Lurching out of his sweat soiled bed, Giddeon staggered lifelessly to the bathroom. Feeling around in the dark, the mournful man found and flicked on the dim light that hovered over the sink. He stared into the streaked mirror at the pathetic reflection that glared hatefully back at him.

The guilt he still carried deep within after all this time was too much for him to keep bottled up, and he couldn't bear the weight of it any longer. He should've done something then, helped them. He should have tried to fight back. Instead, he just stood there and watched as his parents were butchered. Giddeon lowered his head, disgusted by the worthless man in the mirror exposing him for the coward he knew he truly was inside.

Deep down, the defeated shell he had become was tired of living like this. Giddeon didn't want to wander through his meaningless existence anymore. Gripping the sink, he gritted his teeth with punishing pressure. There wasn't a point to any of it anymore. Everyone would be better off without a piece of shit like him, poisoning everything he touched. He was just a cancer that spread his wickedness, sorrow, and pain onto everyone else. He was weak. He was disgusting.

It took one fleeting thought: *What would my parents think if they saw me now? Witnessed all the vile things I've done?* Giddeon hung his head in anguish, not able to look at himself any longer. Spotting one of Dominick's discarded razor blades on the counter, he reached out and picked it up. The beast within him surged to the forefront, urging him on. The burning, tingling need crawled across his skin like a thousand spiders.

Deprived of any rational thinking, his fingers skillfully dismantled the razor. Without a moment's pause or hesitation, Giddeon dragged the sharp edge of his salvation along the inside of his already marked up arm. It sank deep into his sweaty flesh, and the blessed sting thankfully brought an exultant calm over him. The sudden rush of euphoria flooded is system, erased his self-hate, all of his guilt, and thawed his cold heart enough so that he finally *felt...* human again. The gratifying ache distracted him from his soul crushing reality.

But, that sensation was short lived. The pleasure gradually ebbed away, bringing with it the emotionally crippling sorrow he tried so hard to drown out.

Unsatisfied with his brief reprieve from reality, Giddeon pressed harder the second time. It elicited a recharging sting that jump-started his dead nerves, awakening all of his senses. A throaty groan ripped from his trembling lips. Still teetering on the edge of pleasure and pain, he dug deeper still. His arm burned as if it'd been set on fire as the blissfully excruciating pain traveled down his limb. He reveled in each new shockwave of sensation, like an addict experiencing his first high. Unleashing a moan of ecstasy, the sick man plunged the blade in farther, flaying his willing flesh wide open. He glanced down at himself when the sound of trickling made its way into his consciousness, and noticed for the first time the dark wet surface and his wet sticky fingers.

"WHAT THE FUCK!" Dominick screamed in abhorrence as he rushed in the small bathroom, turning on the main light switch. Giddeon blinked rapidly as the brilliant light stole away his sight. The moment his eyes adjusted, he cast them down to where Dominick stared on in horror. Awestruck at the scene laid out before him, he grasped the extent of the damage he'd caused. The sink and floor were covered in blood... his blood. It poured down his arm and into a dark puddle that collected around his feet.

Shit.

"WHAT THE FUCK IS WRONG WITH YOU?" Dominick sprinted out the door, returning a split second later with a thick, navy blue towel. He wrapped Giddeon's shredded arm and applied pressure. Dominick looked all over him with *that* look, the look everyone gave when he was caught self-harming.

Great. I fucked up... big-time, Giddeon thought to himself as Dominick worked on him. He was going to fuck

64

up his one and only shot at finishing his search... his need for justice and revenge, destroyed by his moment of weakness. Giddeon was going to have to stop being a depressing pussy long enough to get his shit together, focus, and man-up.

Shaking his head at him, Dominick didn't look pissed; he looked concerned for a fuck-up like him. Weird. The detective's face was ashen gray in color. Giddeon really must've scared the shit out of him.

"I'm... I'm sorry. It won't happen again." Giddeon refrained from saying more. He couldn't promise him that. It just wasn't true. "Not while you let me stay here," he quickly amended.

Dominick's voice softened its previous harshness. "Giddeon..."

But the defeated man just shook his head in warning. "Don't, Detective."

Dominick glared at him for what seemed like forever, then finally spoke up. "This. Can't. Happen. This *won't* happen. Anymore. You need help. This..." He motioned with his hand at the disturbing scene around them, painted in Giddeon's blood. "This isn't normal. If you're staying here, and want my help with your parents' case, you'll get some help. Do you understand what I'm telling you? I don't care if it's anger management, addiction, or all of the above. You *will* go. No exceptions. And you start tomorrow."

Giddeon looked at Dominick, broken, defeated, and

utterly wrecked, then nodded his reluctant agreement. After all, he had no other choice. It was very obvious that now was not his time to go. Once again, Giddeon had to refocus his goal and his priorities. His parents. Justice. Revenge.

Eva's face drifted into his mind. She was a straight-to-the-point, bold, no nonsense, and crass woman. His golden Angel had absolutely no fear of him whatsoever. He thought back to the way her eyes roved over him, looking at him the way no woman had ever dared. The intensity of it cracked open a hairline space in his black, lifeless heart.

He would go see her tomorrow. She did say she was an addiction counsellor, and Giddeon definitely had plenty of addictions. For the first time in a very long time, he had something to look forward to that had nothing to do with hurting himself... or someone else. He wasn't sure what to think about that. He'd been numb for so long; there was safety in that... control.

If Giddeon allowed himself to feel again, it'd leave him weak. Vulnerable. That was dangerous. Snapping back to the depressing reality he was in, he finally spoke up. "So, patch me up, Detective. Looks like I have a long day ahead of me tomorrow."

Dominick was already cleaning up the tiled floor. "You're a stupid asshole... you know that, right? I should take you to the hospital, but I know you'd fight me the whole way. And if they admitted you, we'd never get Dalton... or the men who killed your parents. Instead, you'd get a one-way ticket to the nuthouse. I'm acting purely on my selfish need to get the bigger asshole, so if you could just reign in the crazy while we are working, that'd be great."

"I hear you. I'll go tomorrow and talk about my feelings and shit. Whatever it takes. I've got to finish this. It's time they get peace. It's time we all got some peace."

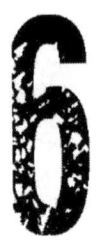

Portree Harbor,
Isle of Skye,
Scotland

"Honestly, Behr, you don't have to stay here to clean. I can handle this mess. I've done renovation projects dozens of times. I'm a big, tough girl. I got this." Ellora flexed her muscles, playing around, trying to prove her point. "Besides, Gavin's going to kill you if you take any more days off work."

Behr continued to gather up all the broken glass and debris, shaking his head in disagreement. "It's the least I can do, love. If it weren't for my explosive anger, and my less than graceful entrance, this place wouldnae nearly be as trashed as it is now." Ellora laughed as he finished his statement.

"And the understatement of the year award goes to… the Incredible Hulk!" Giggling, she looked over at Behr's face as she mocked him bursting through the windows and crouching down on the littered ground, striking a manly pose. Behr dropped what he was doing and stalked over to his raven-haired beauty. Wrapping his large, muscular arms around her waist from behind, he tugged her into him and whispered in her ear. "Helping clean up the mess I left behind is the least I can do… It's what I should be doing, love. Gavin and everyone else is behind you one-hundred percent. They all want to help you see this through."

Ellora turned into his solid body. Wrapping her arms around his neck, she pulled him closer and insisted half-heartedly, "Really, Behr, you can go… I got this." She meant what she said, but she still didn't want him to go. She could melt into the warmth of his body and stay that way all day. But, that was exactly the problem. Whenever he left, it was as though Behr took a big piece of her with him. When he did, she experienced an overwhelming emptiness in the pit of her stomach that ached until they found their way back to each other. She suffered actual pain when they were separated.

Nibbling her way up the side of his thick tanned neck, Ellora made it to his earlobe and softly sucked on the tender skin. She was rewarded with exactly the response she was expecting… A deep rumbling groan vibrated out of his massive chest.

"Aaaaah, Ellora. You are driving me mad, woman. You donnae really want me to leave, do ya, love?" Ellora shook her head, rubbing her face slowly against his neck as she did. Cradling his face in her hands, she pressed her lips to his fervently.

In her ambitious state, Ellora didn't hold back. She dove right in, tilting her head for better access as she sought to deepen the kiss. Her tongue explored his hot, expectant mouth. Behr growled roughly as he gripped a fistful of her shirt, and Ellora couldn't help but smile. He was losing his grip on his control, his muscles flexing and twitching from the stress of holding back. But, she didn't want him to. She wanted him to let go.

Daringly, she locked her leg around his hip, and when she pulled him in tighter, Behr finally reacted. Reaching up, he grabbed hold of the elastic holding her hair up and yanked it out. Behr couldn't wait any longer. He ran his hands through the silky strands, gently pulling her head where he wanted it. Strong lips crashed down on hers with a desperate need to possess. His movements became dominant and demanding, pushing the kiss deeper. All that could be heard was their panting breaths mingling together in the silent warehouse. The sound echoed around them, heightening their need for each other.

Ellora willingly gave herself over to Behr as he sought to devour her. Pushing his tongue past the seal of her lips, he stroked hers with intoxicating friction that drove her wild. Without warning, he untangled his hands from her hair and wrapped them behind the backs of her thighs. He brought her legs off the ground, effortlessly lifting her in the air. She reflexively wrapped her tiny legs around his solid steel waist.

Behr groaned out against her whetted lips, "Yes, my love, I want to feel your warmth wrapped all 'round me." He worshiped her with his attentive mouth. Each tender touch and glide of his expert tongue had her climbing higher and higher, needing a release. From what, she wasn't sure of yet. Ellora coiled her hands in his thick, dark hair, tugging him impossibly closer.

"Behr… I Love you. So much."

After her quiet admission, Ellora swayed with the rhythm from each commanding step Behr took, moving with purposeful steps across the room. A breeze created by the swiftness of his stride tickled the back of her neck. Her back met the cracked stucco wall moments later, and a wave of exhilaration flooded Ellora as he pressed his weight into her, caging her in.

A breathy moan escaped her lips the moment Behr's body pressed into her. Ellora submitted herself to the beautiful pressure he created as he deliberately ground his hips against hers in a rhythm that was soon to be her undoing. For the first time, neither one of them stopped. They desperately needed to be closer to each other. Their bodies called out to one another, needing to feel skin against skin. No matter how close they got, it was never close enough. They always wanted more… needed more.

Ellora's breathing grew ragged as his strong, roughened fingers dug into her thighs, massaging the flesh of her quivering legs. Her skin grew hot under the provocative path of his possessive touch. Ellora was surprised at where her thoughts were headed, because she desperately longed for his demanding hands to continue their torturous pressure further up her thighs where her ache was growing more and more powerful.

"I love you, Ellora. You. Are. Mine. Always," he proclaimed against her throat as he dragged his lips down the length of her neck. His stubble abraded her heated flesh and sent shivers down her spine.

Loud cat-calling and whistling had them snapping their heads up and over to the door. There stood Gavin and Adelle, wiggling their eyebrows and smiling at the hot couple. Ellora wasn't sure how long they'd been standing there, but the pair looked *very* entertained by the free show they unknowingly provided. Not quite ready to let go, Behr continued to place wet kisses over her cheeks, chin, forehead, the tip of her nose, and both eyelids. He was completely undeterred by their invading company.

"Ugh!" Ellora groaned in frustration, "We've got to start doing this in private. We are always getting interrupted... right when things start getting good." Pouting up at her very own dreamy alpha male, she jutted her bottom lip out like a petulant child. Behr nibbled the protruding lip she offered, slowly lowering her back down to the ground. Once the dazed girl's feet touched the dirty concrete floor, reality set in. Ellora flushed scarlet at her very brazen, public act.

Behr ran his thumb over her reddened cheeks. Nuzzling into the hair beside her neck, he whispered low in her ear, lacing his tone thick with the lust he tried so hard to keep at bay, "Soon, love. Very soon, I will have you all to myself. And I promise you, no one will interrupt us." She gasped in surprise as he growled his own frustrations and bit her neck. Excitement and anticipation for time alone with Behr had her trembling all over. She couldn't wait for that promise to come to fruition.

Adelle tip-toed carefully through the debris, trying hard to avoid the dirtiest spots. She cautiously avoided the glass littered all over the floor. "You are never going to get this place up and running if you spend all of your time necking on every surface and in every room available, you know. You two can christen the place with your love when it's all done up proper." Avoiding a low hanging cobweb, Adelle ducked and squeaked out, "Eeeew. It's so dirty and disgusting in here! How is this even romantic?"

Gavin swiped the cobweb out of the way. Grasping her elbow, he turned her around to face him. "C'mon, Ellie... It doesnae hurt to get a little dirty... yeah?" Ellora smiled at them as he wiggled his brows, winking at her naughtily.

Adelle just rolled her eyes at his innuendo. "Aye, stop that!" She giggled when the beautiful man before her wiped his finger in a pile of dust and brushed it down the porcelain skin of her bare arm.

"Not so fast, pretty boy. Before this girl gets down and

dirty with anyone, she expects to be wined and dined first."
Turning on her heel, Adelle crossed her arms over her chest
stubbornly. She left his side and walked toward her friend.
Gavin absentmindedly nodded his head. His serious
expression looked as if he was taking mental notes and filing
them away for later.

He adored her so much. Ellora looked on, hoping that
Adelle would get over the past and give Gavin a chance to
prove he'd changed his playboy ways. After all, neither one
of them were kids anymore. Ellora took in a few calming
breaths, attempting to douse the passion that Behr had
ignited. She looked up, feeling him watch her intently. His
eyes were dilated fully, blocking out the blue of his irises.
Grudgingly, he let her go. Still hot and bothered, she
stumbled on quivering legs a total of two steps before he
grabbed hold of her hand, stopping her in her tracks.

Behr walked right up to her with a devilish glint in his
eyes. His large, imposing frame towered over hers.
Smirking, he bent low, like a gentleman greeting his lady. He
lowered his lips to her knuckles and pressed a soft kiss,
promising a 'to be continued' with his eyes. Ellora's stomach
flipped and clenched tight in response to his touch, the soft
kiss, and the look that roved over her.

Reluctantly, she pulled away from him. If she didn't
get back to work, this place would never be ready... not
anytime soon. Clapping her hands together, she psyched
herself up for the job ahead. It was time to get down to

business. "All right, guys. No more fooling around." She looked right at Behr, who smiled broadly at her. Oh, this boy. That smile could melt the clothes off a nun. "Let's get down to work. Gavin, hand me the wide broom and dust pan. Behr... please grab the large garbage can over by the back door. Time to get this stuff off the floor so we can really get some work done in here."

Adelle interrupted before Ellora could assign her a job. "I brought over snacks from Kristy's." Adelle smiled brilliantly, lightly shaking a large bag dangling from her perfectly manicured fingertips.

"Good, I'm starving."

"Aye, sister, you're starving a'right... But, it's for that man over there, I'd say." She nodded her head in Behr's direction, scrunching up her nose as she teased the flush-faced girl. Ellora's wide, embarrassed smile was her only answer. Brat!

"All right, Miss Hollywood Glamour, I have a change of clothes for you." Pointing a threatening finger in the fashionable girl's direction, she continued, "You, *Miss Thang*... owe me a day of labor, and I'm collecting that debt today." The dressed to the nine, strawberry-haired princess grabbed the clothes she was handed and stuck her tongue out as she strutted into the decrepit bathroom to change.

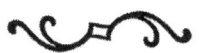

Dalton remained motionless, his sharp eyes transfixed on the monitor in front of him. The brilliant light from the sizable screen was the only illumination in the otherwise dark room he occupied. The soft glow wrapped around him and faded away. His chin rested on his steepled fingers as he sat glaring with disdain. It took all of his willpower to keep his demeanor controlled and calm. He wanted nothing more than to jump through the monitor when that Neanderthal put his hands all over *his* dark beauty. It should be his lips tasting her. No one else was deserving.

The only thing that kept him from making his presence known was that he knew he was no match, physically, against that big beast hanging all over her. This was a game of chess. He had to choose his moves wisely. Dalton sneered as Ellora swept up the mess around her. "I'm going to have to work quicker than I had originally anticipated. I had no idea you were this desperate for affection, my love." Dalton spoke to the object of his deepest obsession while he stroked his fingertips over her hair on the screen.

It was easy enough to find out who the previous owners of the warehouse were, and he knew full well his green-eyed goddess wouldn't be able to resist a family business, or a cheap lease. Dalton had installed several hidden monitors a week before she signed the contract. Now, he could keep an intimate eye on her, learn what she liked and what she didn't. He enjoyed appraising her every move.

The months she spent away from him nearly drove him mad. That was time he was determined to make up for. "You'll be mine soon enough, Ellora Belle, and this time, I won't let you go. You belong to me. Since the moment I laid my eyes on you… You. Were. Mine. In due time, I will own all of you. Mind. Body. And soul." Kissing his fingers, Dalton pressed them firmly over Ellora's stunning face, just as she seemed to look directly at him on the screen. "I will possess all of you."

Pulling out his cell, Dalton confidently punched in the numbers he had previously been given and waited. He wasn't sure until now, but he was going to have to switch tactics. Time was of the essence, and he had to up his game.

"Shannon? Hello, darling. I was told by an associate of mine about your situation. Well, I believe we can help each other out. Yes. We both have something the other needs. Let's meet up and discuss it. Tell me your address. I will have my man contact you when I'm ready to collect you."

Dalton ended the call without any confirmation from the girl. She didn't know it yet, but her choices had officially ended. She was caught up in Dalton's web, and just like the rest of his 'employees', she wouldn't ever get out. Sitting back down in his chair, his eyes immediately located Ellora on one of the many monitors set up. The enigmatically disturbed man glared, infatuated with the one girl who had ever dared tell him no.

She was working herself into a sweat. He despised the idea of *his* girl getting her hands dirty. She deserved better. She deserved to be indulged and waited on hand and foot, not the other way around. She deserved riches, power, and status. She deserved to be in the presence of Dalton, and he would have her soon enough. Whether she chose to ignore that truth or not was no matter. That was a lesson she'd learn soon enough.

Being this close to his green-eyed temptress, and not at liberty to stroke her perfect skin, was driving him insane with months of pent up desire. He desperately wanted to be in a room alone with her. It became quite clear to Dalton from the very first week he arrived that he was going to have to get rid of Ellora's new… admirer, and fast. If he waited too long, she would most certainly be tainted by the big man pushing his way into her arms, and most obviously, into her bed. Dalton wanted to get his hands on her first.

Many sleepless nights, Dalton fantasized about being the one and only man who got to break her in. There was no way this beast was going to be that man. He already had several back up plans lined up for getting this bearded brute out of the way. Permanently. There was no changing his mind… No one touched what was his and lived. No one ever had, and no one ever would.

7

Eva looked out over the tight-fitting, crowded circle of chairs. She was a little shocked when she caught sight of Giddeon hovering by the entrance, hesitating by the heavy metal door. It looked as though he was going to bolt at any moment. Obviously, he was completely out of his comfort zone here. The thought made her smile. He didn't look like the man trying hard to scare and intimidate, like he'd done when she first met him. He just looked lost.

Giddeon scanned the room. His eyes connected, locking in on hers. They regarded each other for a few more silent moments, the tension rising noticeably. Slowly... very slowly, he willed his legs to move forward, inching his way across the room. All of his focus was on the beautiful blonde, Eva. Was it possible that she had become even more stunning since he last feasted his eyes on her? The room and all the people in it ceased to exist as he made his way over to his Angel. Staring at nothing else around him, his eyes were imprisoned by hers.

The expression that was ever-present on his face gave her pause as he approached. The counsellor's stomach twisted itself into knots when the powerful pull from his dark onyx eyes were cast down on her.

He was dangerous. Not just biker bad boy dangerous… he was *really* a force to be reckoned with. She could see it in his unusually cold eyes, void of any emotion. That is, until he aimed them in her direction. She didn't dare put a name to the look he struck her with.

Which was exactly why she had to try and stay away from him. Getting too close to a person like him was bad for Eva. She was having a hard enough time trying to keep her own life on track. Warning bells sounded off inside of her every time he was around, and she knew that Giddeon would drag her down into the darkness with him. After all, misery craved company. She'd experienced that first-hand growing up.

Dark and marked up, Eva knew he had been through the ringer, she just didn't know what happened… yet. But, she would get to the bottom of it. Instinctively, she wanted to reach out and help him, help end the suffering he tried so hard to hide. That suffering, she recognized it all too well, and she would help him start fresh and enjoy living his life.

It would be extremely difficult to avoid him now that he would be in her group sessions. Detective Antonelli called her early that morning and gave a *very* brief overview of Giddeon's story. Story… Yeah, right. He told her he had issues and tragedies that he had suffered as a kid, but gave no specifics. When she offered other groups available, besides hers, the Detective said Giddeon refused every other session... He specifically requested her.

When Eva asked why the sudden urgency, Dominick touched briefly on what had happened last night. Giddeon was a cutter. Oh, yeah, and the best part... he had a terrible anger problem as well. Great. Eva asked him to elaborate, but he said he wasn't at liberty to disclose it. Eva's curiosity was definitely piqued. What was the deal with this dark stranger?

He made his way through the circle of chairs with ease, as his sinister, ominous presence and marked up body parted the group like the Red Sea, all too eager to move out of his way. Giddeon stood next to Eva, shooting daggers at the man who currently occupied the chair next to her. Jeff, a man struggling terribly to kick a meth habit, twitched anxiously as the nefarious figure towered over him. Jeff looked everywhere but up at the menacing stranger.

"You're sitting in *my* seat. Get up... Now."

Jeff, not willing to pick a fight with a man who looked like he could be the Grimm Reaper himself, got up swiftly. The moment the chair was free, Giddeon grabbed the back of it and dragged it closer to Eva. Jeff nervously scratched at one of the many scabs on his arm, muttering under his breath when he was at a safe distance away, "Whatever. Prick."

Oh, God, please keep me strong. I have to stay away from this dangerously delicious man, Eva silently pleaded to herself.

"Morning, Angel."

Eva rolled her eyes at his insistence on calling her that. She couldn't help but ask, "What are you doing here? There are other groups, other counsellors."

He cocked his head to the side and flashed a self-assured, crooked smirk in her direction. His goal was to look confident, in control, but Eva could see right through him.

"I'm here to see you."

She had seen this many, many times before. He wasn't there to just flirt, or try to pick her up. He was there for a real reason and was struggling to keep that reason hidden. He needed help, just like everyone else in the group. But, there was something about this man that pulled her into his world. He was somehow different than all the other cases she'd seen or heard of.

Giddeon's destructive personality mirrored that of a dark tornado, all-consuming and undeniably lethal. Instead of running in the other direction, like most seemed to do when encountering him, Eva was unfathomably drawn directly into the path of his destruction. The longer she was in his presence, the stronger the pull. She shook her head to free her wayward thoughts. He was already getting inside of her head, and he'd only uttered seven words total.

"Okay, guys, time to start. My name is Evangelina Baker. Please, everyone, call me Eva. I'm a survivor of the domestic and substance abuse I suffered at the hands of my mother and step-father. I am your counsellor and group leader."

Everyone answered back mechanically through sheer habit, "Hi, Eva."

All except Giddeon. She could feel him watching her every move from her peripheral vision. She snuck a quick glance in his direction, only turning her head slightly. His eyes were hyper-focused, penetrating, and infinitely intense. "Pleasure to meet you, Angel." His voice came out sounding irresistibly low and rough, like sharp gravel. It did strange things in the pit of her stomach.

Eva didn't like the way he used her nickname. Unlike the loving way her grandparents made it sound, the way Giddeon rolled the syllables off his tongue sounded uncomfortably familiar, intimate, and a little dirty. He had a way of manipulating her emotions. The way his tongue caressed the words as they left his mouth had Eva blushing as though she was put on display before him, completely naked and vulnerable.

She dove right into the meeting, trying hard to ignore the powerful affect he was drawing out of her. The greetings and brief synopses of why each member was there started. They all took turns around the circle. Eva had heard them all before. None of them were new members, so she tuned them out. Everyone except, of course, for Giddeon. Her ears perked up when it was his turn, curiosity getting the better of her.

Taking an exaggerated pull of air and blowing it out

with forceful exacerbation, the reluctant man spoke up. "My name's Giddeon, and I'm addicted to pain." The words dripped with ecstasy as they passed through his lips. His tone dipped to a lower octave as he voiced the word 'pain'. Like just speaking the word gave him pleasure.

"To yourself... or to others?" one of the other group members asked before Eva was able to ask aloud. Giddeon turned his black eyes on him. The weight of his stare had the other man shifting his gaze away like a submissive dog. Eva thought that was what Giddeon wanted... To show his dominance. To elicit fear.

"Both," he answered, with no further explanation as to why. What was the deal with this guy?

Group was very intense this week. Eva was pretty sure it had something to do with Giddeon's presence. He definitely put everyone else on edge. Adam was an alcoholic and had an anger problem, as well. Both issues triggered one another. He was one of her more difficult personalities to deal with in group. His assignment last week was to sit down with his brothers and ask how his addictions impacted their lives in a negative way. It's good for addicts to hear how destroying others' lives because of their addictions didn't affect them alone.

He was obviously having a hard time coping with the

harsh realities of life without the comfort of alcohol. When she came around to him in the circle and asked if he completed his assignment, he snapped. This wasn't uncommon. People who have addictive personalities are irritable, agitated, and angry at the world. Sobriety is a very rough uphill battle.

So, after all these years, Eva was completely unfazed by the outbursts and tantrums of the group members. After all, she was once in their spot. When she pressed Adam harder, he shouted at her.

"Who the fuck are you to tell me what to do, you stupid bitch? You're not my mom!" He could be a serious prick on his bad days. This was usually about the time when he would get up and head over to the refreshments table for some coffee to cool off.

It all happened so fast. It took the over-worked girl a few seconds to catch up. Giddeon flew at Adam, easily tackling him to the ground.

"Don't. You. *Ever*. Talk to her like that again! You worthless piece of shit!" When Giddeon wrapped his hands around Adam's neck and squeezed, everyone jumped into action. While Adam's eyes were bulging out in a shocked panic, Giddeon had an eerie smile plastered across his face. He seemed too at ease with the fact that he was choking out another human being.

Leaning down close to his face, he hissed, "I have killed before… and for less. I won't hesitate with you…" It took four guys a full minute to pry him off. "I will kill you if you do it again."

Eva sat back, stunned. The hairs on the back of her neck stood on end at his terrifying confession. This guy said he'd killed before. Her gut twisted at the thought, and she wondered if it'd been a true statement or just threats to scare Adam. Her instincts about him when they first met had been correct. Giddeon Cane was dangerous... toxic. If he wasn't careful, he'd end up in prison at the end of this session, if he wasn't already on his way there. Eva knew she'd have to fight to keep her guards up around this unpredictably violent man.

She couldn't tell if it was her sick and twisted nature or a morbid curiosity, but she just had to figure out what had made him like this. And just like that... Giddeon Cane had successfully dug his talons into her... She was hooked.

When riled up, Giddeon looked like a vicious, wild animal, desperate to get out of a trap, as he struggled against the arms of those who held him. He snarled at the men holding him back. "Get your fucking hands off me, or I will cut you up into tiny little pieces." His outburst got the reaction he was looking for—submission and fear. They abruptly let him go. Giddeon took a moment to straighten himself out, then stalked toward Adam... looking to finish what he started.

Eva snapped out of her stupor and jumped up out of her chair to block Giddeon's way, standing directly in his path to Adam. Placing her hands on his chest, she pushed back to keep him at bay, which was incredibly stupid, she knew. This man could easily destroy her. She could, in no way, stop him if he wanted to surge forward. But he did just that. He stopped dead in his tracks and gazed down at her, his nostrils flaring in his angry state. But, he calmed down as he gazed directly into her eyes. Cold chills broke out on the back of her neck and rippled down her spine from the deep, penetrating glare he cast down on her.

After a breathless moment had passed, and the dizzy haze cleared, she remembered that she could talk. "Giddeon. Stop! It's okay. Adam is just having trouble dealing with his sobriety. He doesn't mean any harm."

Giddeon continued his watchful gaze on her as he addressed Adam on the floor behind her. "He shouldn't be talking to you like that, Angel. You are here to help us. He needs to respect that." Her dark destroyer looked around the room at every single person in warning. "You all do."

He dragged his eyes away from the other members and back down on the brave blonde in front of him. The air crackled between them and ignited something deep inside of her. Eva tried to ignore the connection that had passed between them. "It's okay. I'm a big girl. I can take care of myself. I never asked for a dark knight to swoop in here and fight all my battles for me. You are triggering the others. We've all worked really hard to get to the stage we're in right now. I will not tolerate a relapse because you came charging in here, unable to control yourself. Just breathe."

Eva could see Giddeon struggling within himself to do just that. He looked as though he was fighting a battle within himself, like a split personality. He shook with the effort to contain his rage. She cupped his face and lightly tapped his cheek. "Giddeon… just relax." For a fleeting moment, Giddeon's cold eyes warmed to a dark chocolate brown, and his expression softened under her touch. He almost smiled at her. She could see his mouth twitch. She boldly looked right back at him.

When Adam coughed, rubbing his sore throat, just like that, the softness was gone. It passed through him so fast, it was as though it never happened. The murderous rage was back, and it was directed right at Adam.

"Oh my God. Get over yourself already, will ya! We get it. You're a dangerous badass. No one should mess with you. Everyone gets the message, okay. Sit down!" With all of her strength, Eva yanked back on the neckline of Giddeon's shirt as hard as she could, until he fell back heavily into his chair with a loud thud. "Good boy. Stay!"

Turning her attention to Adam, she addressed him quickly. "Listen… Stop being a dick, okay. You obviously triggered the new guy when you spoke to me that way, and it pisses me off when you do that to me anyways. Don't disrespect me, or any woman for that matter. Ever."

Adam hung his head in embarrassed shame. "Look, I'm really sorry, Eva."

Lifting up her hand, she interrupted him, nodding. "I know." She totally understood this. She knew he was struggling. "I forgive you. Let's just forget it and move on."

Adam held out his hand to Giddeon. "I'm sorry, man. We cool?" An utterly disgusted look crossed over Giddeon's face, like Adam had dipped his hand in shit first.

"Ugh, I'm sick of this already! Just shake the man's hand and let's move on."

When Giddeon made no move to make peace, she kicked him fast and hard on the shin. A satisfied smirk curled her lips when he let out a loud grunt. Chuckling heartily, he unexpectedly smiled ear to ear with amusement. Eva was sure she spotted the moment his cold dark eyes sparked to life. Finally, she received a warm, genuine smile from him, but she figured it was only because she brought him pain. Not good.

The brilliance of his perfect white teeth stood out in contrast to his collection of tattoos and scars. Her dark stallion was a magnificent creature. Arching his brow, he nodded at her. Looming over Adam, Giddeon grabbed his hand and shook it tensely. It looked as though he squeezed it a little too hard, because when he let go, Adam shook it out a few times.

"Yeah. We're cool. Never talk to her like that again, and we're cool."

The group took a short fifteen-minute break to grab a snack, smoke break, or coffee. Once everyone sat back down,

Eva started the confessions portion of the session. It was always harder for new comers at first, to reveal terrible things about themselves—who they are, what they've done, or what they were doing. No one wanted to be judged, but venting and listening to others' experiences was healthy. It helped a person recognize the action the next time they were triggered, so they could make an attempt to change their course of action.

Eva started with the person on Giddeon's right side. Going counter clockwise would put her before him in the circle. He would go last. She was anxious to hear his story. She knew his would be a dark one. Giddeon drew her into his world, whether she liked it or not, and she was helpless against the pull. She was hooked and wanted to dig deeper into the man who bulldozed his way into her life.

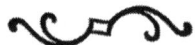

Giddeon couldn't help but stare. His Angel had a brilliant fire burning underneath her golden façade. Once ignited, her flames were all-consuming; he could see them hiding behind her eyes when she was mad. She intrigued him like no one ever had before. This golden beauty had absolutely no fear of him whatsoever. She was bold, handsy, and crass. It was damn near impossible to be in a room with her and not get pulled closer.

His Angel was just like the sun—bright, breathtaking,

and the center of everything. If you got too close to her, you could get burned. All the other human beings there were like her dutiful planets, just orbiting around her faithfully.

Giddeon almost bolted when he first arrived, having second thoughts about participating in group sessions, but when those ocean blues locked on his cold lifeless eyes, she awoke something long dead inside him. Before he knew what was happening, he was moving toward her.

He should've been furious by the way she manhandled him. He was surprised that it didn't make him fly into one of his manic rages. She didn't faze him in that way, though, and instead, quite the opposite happened. Interesting. He had to admit, he loved it. The delicious pain that followed her impressive soccer kick to the shins almost had him come undone in front of everyone.

His golden Angel could give him the two things he needed most... pleasure and pain. The wall around his heart cracked a little more, but like always, Giddeon almost ruined everything when he let the beast loose on that man. He wanted to kill that disgusting scumbag when he called her a bitch, like she was common no-good trash. He still wanted to make him bleed.

Almost immediately, his very dark reality changed when she pressed her delicate hands over his chest. With one touch, she had pulled him out of the darkness he dwelled in for a few precious moments. She had a power over him... over the beast. *That* he couldn't understand or explain. That loss of control scared the shit out of him. Control is all he had that was truly his.

Just one look into her eyes, and all the power he possessed was in her hands. After a much needed break, she had them all sit back down in the depressing circle of regret and failure. Guess this was the part where she had everyone reveal something about themselves. To reveal the cause that led them all there. Great. He was gonna have to sit and listen to all their blubbering bullshit. He wasn't sure if it was like protocol or whatever to have the newbie go last, but that was where he ended up.

Curiosity made him a little anxious as he waited to hear Angel's story. At the beginning of group, she said she was a survivor of domestic and substance abuse at the hands of her parents. A mixture of surprise and abhorrence welled up inside him at the thought of anyone hurting her. She was probably freaked out by him because he just sat back and watched her the whole time. She sat there, trying her best to ignore him while listening to the others.

He was enraptured by the way her perfectly porcelain skin wrinkled as her worry and concern showed for the others. He was enthralled by every move she made... the way she crossed her legs and bounced her foot, an obvious habit of hers. Every change in expression. Every deep breath in lifted her irresistible breasts. Giddeon memorized it all. He memorized her.

Before he knew it, his Angel's turn had arrived.

Giddeon turned his chair around so that he sat facing her and waited. She had his full attention.

Eva fidgeted, nervously twisting her fingers and wringing her hands for a moment. Dipping her head down, she glanced at him through her long feathery eyelashes. Giddeon knew he was probably making her more nervous, staring at her like he was, but his anticipation to hear her glorious voice again made him impatient. Giddeon did his best to force as gentle a smile as he could muster, trying his best to encourage her to go on.

"Well... my mother had always been a heavy drinker. Both of her parents were alcoholics, too. My mother met both my father and step-dad, Rob, in a bar. With my dad, she just drank a lot. But, when my dad tried to quit because of me, my mom was furious. She wasn't ready to stop the partying. It put a wedge between them until my father just had enough one morning. He walked out, just like that. He never came back, not even to see me.

"My mother didn't get into the heavy stuff until she got with Rob. He was into anything that could get him climbing so high, it took days to get back down. He dragged her down to his level because addicts hate to party alone." Eva blew out a shaky breath and bit her lip, concentrating on telling her story.

"The first time I ever got high..." Giddeon's Angel paused and pinched her eyes shut, like recalling the memory was hard to talk about. "I walked into the den, which was an area of the house I was warned never to go into. They were right in the middle of a two-day bender... I think it was meth. I don't really remember. I was curious, jealous, and a little mad as to why they spent so much time and energy on that stuff. They neglected me, forgetting most days to feed me. There were weeks I didn't make it to school. My clothes and shoes were falling apart, but she didn't care anymore. All she cared about was that stuff."

Eva ticked on her fingers all of her mother's offenses. She tried to keep a calm voice, but every other sentence, her voice elevated in anger.

"I walked in on them one day and had had enough, asking, 'What's so good about this stuff, anyway?' Well, Rob thought it would be frickin' hilarious if he forced me to take a 'big girl hit'." Eva wrapped her arms around herself in comfort as she continued the story. "He laughed as he pounced on me, forcing me to the ash-ridden carpet. I tried to fight him off of me, crying out as I struggled to break free from him. I cried out to my mother for help as he easily pinned me down and held me there."

Anger burned its way through Giddeon's veins as he sat and watched Eva shrink in her chair, rubbing her arms as if she could still feel the struggle and the punishing grip from hands that were supposed to protect her. She took in a deep breath to calm herself and continued.

"My mother handed him the needle, smiling the whole time. 'Curiosity killed the cat,' is what Rob whispered in my ear as the needle pierced my arm. They both laughed hysterically when I went limp in his arms from the forced high."

Giddeon watched helplessly as Eva unconsciously scratched and dug at her inner arm, as if she could feel the deadly poison still coursing through her, killing her innocence. He desperately wanted to reach out to her, comfort her, but he didn't really know how.

"My mother, of course, was elated. She clapped excitedly, saying, 'Now that Rob popped your drug cherry, we can party together. Won't that be fun, baby?'" Eva clenched her fists in her lap. "I hated her. So much. And things got worse after that. Rob got meaner toward my mother. She just wasn't hard core enough. They fought constantly. My mother was quick to throw punches. He'd never hit her back, but my mom was very ballsy and knew how to hold her own in a fight, if he ever did. His methods were more emotionally cruel. My hatred grew the more they forced me to party with them."

Eva closed her eyes tight once again and lowered her head in shame, gripping the seat of her chair. Giddeon had to restrain himself from grasping her hands, uncurling them, and lacing his fingers with hers.

"Soon enough, they didn't have to force me. I needed it... wanted it. Badly. It consumed all of my thoughts and dominated all my actions. I hated myself for what I'd become. When I was old enough to fight back, my mother and I got into frequent knock-down, drag-out brawls. This was just pure entertainment for Rob.

"He took an uncomfortable interest in me. It started with him taking my side of the fights. Even if I started, or instigated them, Rob always took my side. This made my mother resent me. When I turned sixteen, her paranoia grew to staggering heights. Rob's interest in me grew as I did. She became cruel where I was concerned. She locked me in my room to keep me out of his sight. I'd be bolted up and barricaded for days at a time."

Giddeon watched as she rhythmically rubbed her jean clad thighs over and over obsessively.

"I stopped wearing shorts in the summer, because if Rob even looked at me a certain way, my mother would punish me for it. Her favorite method was putting her cigarettes out on my thighs." She rubbed harder, feeling the burning memory from her past. Giddeon wanted to wrap his warm Angel in his cold arms and keep her protected. But he was too late to save her from that painful past. He was always too late.

"When my mom's fists couldn't hurt me anymore, she found another way to hurt me… pumping me full of drugs for weeks at a time. Then she'd laugh manically when I suffered through agonizing withdrawals, when she kept the drugs from me. It got so bad at home, I had to make a decision: leave home that night, or stay and slowly die that way. I finally had enough and said, 'Fuck this shit'. Any place was better than home.

"I walked into one of those battered women's shelters. It was a very big step for me. But starting over is easy when you are used to having nothing or no one in the first place."

Eva closed her eyes for a moment. Her face lifted up to the ceiling. It looked like she was silently praying. Everyone in the circle was one-hundred percent completely engulfed in her story. She affected everyone around her; Giddeon wasn't the only one.

"It felt amazing to finally have freedom and control over my own life. It's like, with that freedom, I could finally feel what it was like to start living. I was brought to group sessions here by one of the counsellors there. But, like everything else in my life, I struggled to quit. And, once I quit, I struggled to stay sober. It has always been a constant battle to tamp down the beast that's hiding deep inside me, waiting to break free. Waiting for its next fix."

Giddeon's mind snapped to attention at her words. His Angel also struggled with a beast. *This is very interesting.*

"I've been sober for twenty-six months now with no relapses. I used to think hope was unreachable, dangerous to want. That is, until someone offered me their help. They gave me a chance at a normal life and showed me there was another way. There is always another choice that can take you in a completely different direction than where you were headed. You just have to have the strength to reach for it. Now, I hold on to hope. It's as important to me as the air I breathe."

Giddeon couldn't wrap his head around a parent... a mother especially, dragging her daughter into hell with her, just so she wouldn't suffer alone. A mother is supposed to shield and protect their child, no matter the cost. It infuriated him. If he ever came face to face with that woman and... "Did your step-father... did Rob... force himself... on you?" Giddeon wasn't sure where those words came from, or how they left his mouth on their own.

Eva's eyes widened into two enormous saucers, surprised by the gall he had to ask her such a question, and because he broke the protocol of listening only. Her mouth opened and shut several times, knocked completely off guard. Her silence had Giddeon's gut twisting and turning itself into knots. The longer she sat quiet, the more he *had* to know. "Please, Angel. Please, tell me..."

"No! Oh, God, no! My mother would've cut him up into tiny pieces and ate them before she'd have let that happen. She was far too jealous of a person. No. Thankfully, I never had to endure that kind of hell."

Air he wasn't aware he was holding rushed out of his lungs forcefully, easing his worried discomfort. All he could do was nod, grateful for that tiny miracle. He had no words. If anyone ever touched his Angel, he would tear the flesh right off their bones.

All he could do was sit and stare at her. He really admired her. No, he was in awe of her. She was far braver than Giddeon was at that age. His beautiful Angel had a magnificent inner strength that he wished he possessed.

The group sat in a deafening silence, waiting for something. He wasn't sure what. Eva sat picking at the loose threads hanging at the hemline of her shirt. Her mind was still stuck in her painful past. One more cleansing breath later, she picked up her head. Meeting his gaze head on, she took Giddeon's breath away. She was mesmerizing.

For several uninterrupted moments, they stared at one another. The rest of the world fell away; all that remained was the broken monster and his guardian Angel. Her gaze never faltered as she continued to search his eyes. For the first time in his life, he wondered what she thought of when she looked at him.

Giddeon watched in fascination as her pink tongue darted out to wet her dry lips. He fixated on the movement, daydreaming about what her lips would taste like if he ran his tongue along its seam and how her plump lips would feel pressed against his.

He was brought out of his pleasurable daydream and back to the present when the girl in question, not so subtly, cleared her throat. Those thoughts... Where the hell had they come from? He must have been losing his mind. Shaking his head, he hoped it'd shake out those wayward thoughts as well. He ran his hands through his mess of hair, repeating the motion several times, getting the courage to look back at her.

With an arched brow, she slowly cocked her head to the side. A smirk grew steadily before turning into a full blown smile, tempting Giddeon... drawing him to her. She was killing him. He'd have given anything to climb inside that head of hers. What was she thinking about?

"Giddeon... It's your turn."

Oh... *Shit.*

Eva spoke up. "What led you here to me?" She faltered, catching her slip on words. Giddeon's eyes dilated, catching sight of her growing blush. *This is very interesting indeed.*

"I mean, what led you here... to us, that is?"

Shit! Talk about a mood damper. He didn't want to talk about his shitty, fucked up life. He wanted to take her into an empty room and find *other* things to do with their time.

"That's a very loaded question, Angel. I'm not sure I can answer that." Giddeon watched as her eyebrows pinched together in a cute mixture of confusion and curiosity. Eva was trying just as hard to figure him out, as he was trying to figure her out.

"Well, what was the *cause* that led you to your...umm, addiction?" Eva hoped that he would open up. She was dying to find out more about this mysterious and dangerous man. She doubted that she'd get much out of him, but she was determined to find out. No matter how many sessions it took, she *would* find out more.

Giddeon rubbed the back of his neck up and down several times, over and over. "Shit! I don't know where to begin." Eva leaned in closer to him, giving him her undivided attention. The dark, broken man struggled to think with the smell of his Angel's intoxicating perfume wafting over and wrapping itself around him.

"The... cause..." He caught himself repeating the words out loud as his mind cast him back into the darkest part of his past. Countless moments ticked by before he was able to open his mouth again. "I... I watched as my parents were brutally butchered to death."

Eva gasped in shock. "Where were you, Giddeon, when it happened?" The emotionally checked-out man almost didn't hear her question. It came out soft and quietly. Everyone in the circle was quiet. You could've heard a pin drop as they waited to hear more. No one dared look at him, though; they kept their eyes on the floor.

Giddeon didn't want their sorrow or their pity. Irritation bubbled up to the surface. He shook his head and brought his thumbs to his temples, pressing the pressure point roughly and concentrating hard on not letting his anger take over. He didn't want to flip the fuck out. Not again. Not in front of his Angel. If they thought what he'd done to Adam earlier was bad, they definitely didn't want to be in the same room with him when the beast came out to play.

His chest heaved as air rushed in and out of his lungs in rapid succession. He couldn't seem to get enough air. He couldn't breathe in this tight space, drowning in the stale air in the cramped room. If he didn't get a grip on himself soon, the all too familiar darkness would cloud over his vision and do something he'd regret later.

Giddeon leapt out of his chair, abruptly standing. The overly aggressive movement caused his chair to crash to the ground. He had to get out of there. He kicked his chair out of the way so he could leave the tight circle without ramming right through another person.

"Wait, Giddeon. It's okay. We'll only go as far as *you* want to." Eva reached out and grabbed his forearm to stop his retreat.

Yanking his arm away from her with unnecessary force, he roared out so loud the walls vibrated. "Don't fucking touch me!" He didn't mean to lash out at her. She was the very last person he wanted that to happen to. But, when that need to hurt someone clawed its way out of his black soul to find its next victim, it was over for the unfortunate person standing too close to him.

He couldn't let that happen to Eva. He wouldn't. Taking a chance, he glanced over his shoulder at her. She wasn't scared. He shook his head at her. She should be scared. Hurt showed in her eyes at his outburst, though she tried hard to hide the useless emotion behind a hard front.

Giddeon softened his voice. "Just don't touch me. Not right now. Okay?" The dark man struggled to take a breath in. He had hurt her, and it twisted at his gut, sickening him.

The need to comfort her and the sickness inside of him were conflicting emotions, warring inside of him. But, his need to keep from harming her won out. "It's not you. I just... need a moment to get myself together. Okay, Angel?" He was surprised by how gentle his voice came out sounding.

Nodding silently, Eva's expression changed immediately. She understood. After a few minutes of concentrating on his Angel, the red veil of anger that clouded his vision subsided. She had gently tugged him toward his chair by the arm. This time, Eva turned her chair around to face Giddeon in much the same way he had done to her. They sat so close, their knees touched as they faced one another.

Leaning forward, Eva rested her elbows on her knees, capturing Giddeon with her expressive eyes, pleading with him to go on. "How old were you... when it happened?" His beautiful Angel's voice was laced thick with heavy emotion. Her unique eyes glistened with unshed tears.

"Stop! Don't you *dare* feel bad for me, Angel. I'm not..." Giddeon hesitated for a moment before moving on. "I've done terrible, unspeakable things... I'm a monster." Eva had to know what he was, and he would be up front with her. She deserved it.

Eva scrunched her eyebrows at his speech. Whatever he'd done, he definitely wasn't proud of it. By the broken and lost expression in his eyes, she could tell he had a world of regrets hanging over him. Plaguing him. He definitely wasn't as heartless and hard as he wanted everyone here to see him as. There was more. Deep down, Eva could see that there was more. She just had to find it and pull it out of him.

The determined girl shook her head and huffed at him. She flung her arms out to the sides in frustration. "Take a good look around you, Giddeon! We've all done terrible, unbelievably unfathomable things." Giddeon blinked at her statement. He slowly took a good look around the room at the rough, weary, long-suffering eyes of the afflicted members sitting around him.

He realized that this group probably understood his need more than anyone else. He'd never tell them the depth of his depravity or the lengths he'd go to unleash it. But they were the closest to understanding the *beast* that resided within him.

"I was six years old. I was left standing in a pool of their blood."

Eva let out a pained moan. Closing her eyes, she pinched the bridge of her nose.

He didn't like this look on her face. He definitely didn't deserve her concern. Before she could ask another question, Giddeon lifted his hand to put a stop to it. "That's enough. I'm done."

"Okay." She nodded, immediately agreeing with him. She obviously didn't want to push him any farther. "That's fine, Giddeon. It's your story to tell. Thank you for sharing it with me... us." Everyone in the circle mumbled their thanks out of repetitious habit. Giddeon's heart constricted when Eva finally broke their eye contact, and she looked around at the other group members.

"All right, your homework this week is to reflect about what you could've done differently to change your path. Be ready to share your thoughts. Take care of yourselves. I'll see you all next session."

Giddeon turned his back, ready to run his ass the hell out of that tiny room, relieved that it was finally over. He definitely could use a stiff drink right about then. He was almost to the exit door when a warm, delicate hand wrapped around his bicep, stopping him short. The point of contact had him hissing out a pent up breath as an electric current ran up his arm and down his spine. Shivers trickled through his extremities, heightening his senses.

The dark and disturbed man mumbled under his breath, "You're killing me, sweetheart." He glanced over his shoulder at the golden Angel who had completely mesmerized him.

She lifted one eyebrow at his expression. "You're not planning on bolting on me and never coming back... are you?" She looked concerned as she asked this.

An overpowering feeling came over him; he didn't

want to let her down, but he couldn't promise her that. Slowly, he shook his head, and his mouth spoke against his will. "From you?" Giddeon turned into her, and stepping closer, he looked over her longingly. "How could I run from my guardian Angel?"

Eva took a not so subtle step back, dropping her hand to break their heated point of contact, and swallowed hard. She had to be more careful around him. He was so unpredictable, and she had to keep her guard up. "Do you have a minute?" Her voice broke.

Curling his finger around a perfectly golden lock of hair, he tucked it neatly behind her ear. A tiny gasp escaped, and she bit her lip, trying to hold back the noise. That tiny response awoke the dominant predator in Giddeon. He made her nervous. He had affected her. Now that he knew how, he planned on doing it more often. It wasn't fear that affected her... It was charm and physical connection.

Just as he was starting to feel like a suave Casanova, she smacked his hand away, annoyed. There was his feisty girl. He didn't imagine it, and even with her attitude, it was obvious that he had gotten to her. Even if for the briefest of moments... She was struck by the powerful connection between them, too. Giddeon enjoyed a good chase. Challenge accepted.

"Look, I know you had a rough start today, but I would like to see you next week... In group, I mean. Okay? Keep coming. It'll help, and it *will* get easier. I promise."

Yeah, right. If she only knew him. Giddeon stalked forward until they were touching chest to chest, forcing her to take several steps back lest he plow through her tiny frame. She stopped only when her back hit the wall.

Anger flashed through her fiery eyes, like a ferocious little wild cat. Eva didn't like being cornered. Giddeon lifted her chin up so he could see her eyes.

"You shouldn't make promises you can't keep. You can't help me. No one can." He abruptly let her go, turning on his heel, and once again, headed for the door.

She shouted at his retreating back, "Will you be back?"

Without looking back, Giddeon answered, "I will be back... for you, Angel."

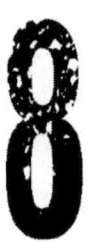

alton pulled his black Maybach S600 up to a small house on Coolin Hills, where he sat with it idling on the side of the road. His driver waited in silence for a minute before turning in his seat to announce the obvious. "We have arrived, Mr. Claiborne. Would you like me to go fetch her for you?" Taking out his cell phone, Dalton completely ignored the man and placed a phone call to his most trusted inside man. He had used this man in the past and knew him to be ruthless, loyal, and reliable.

Enjoying the look on the face of his driver, he made him wait for an answer. "No. Make her wait." He shifted his focus back to the man at the other end of the line once he picked up. "It's me. Where are you at?"

The voice on the other end hesitated before answering, and Dalton could tell by the man's silence that he wasn't going to like what he told him next. "Mr. Claiborne, sir... they are here. They've come back and already stopped by the apartment and Saint Joe's."

Dalton shouted his frustrations, "What do you mean... *they*? Giddeon is in the custody of the Scottish authorities, is he not?" He was becoming more and more fed up with all the incompetence that seemed to surround him. Must he handle everything on his own?

Completely unfazed by Dalton's outburst, his informant continued. "No, sir. Giddeon is here, in the States, and working with the detective. He is staying at his place."

His jaw ticked with his growing frustration. "Really? They've managed to arrive faster than I anticipated. Were you able to clear out Giddeon's place, as I asked?"

The man blew out a breath of his own in frustration, crackling the speakers. "He arrived as I was finishing up. I had to bolt out the back door when he and the detective unexpectedly busted through the front door. I did manage to clear out almost everything and wiped the place down. Giddeon left with the detective soon after they arrived. They didn't stay long."

Dalton pinched the bridge of his nose as he thought about his two angry and determined enemies, who were hell bent on destroying everything he'd worked so hard for. He wasn't sure how much they knew, or how close they were to finding out what was going on.

"That will pose a problem for you. Giddeon is one person you should worry about. He is ruthless, has no sympathy and absolutely no fear. Do. Not. Underestimate him. If I know Giddeon, he will be relentlessly and tirelessly working toward his pursuit to find me. Watch your back at all costs from here on out. Same goes for the detective—he is smart. Don't let him catch you where you aren't supposed to be. He will figure you out."

Dalton could tell his employee was affronted by the tone in his voice, at his praise of Giddeon's skill. Moving on, he asked another question. "How is that girl? Vicky, is it?"

The man answered quickly. "Yes, sir. She's in a coma. She will not come out of it... not alive, anyway. I'll see to that."

Impatience got the best of Dalton as he lashed out at the man once again. "Just finish the job like you were supposed to do from the beginning."

"I will, sir. I would've already, but there's this attendant at the hospital who keeps getting in my way of completing the job. This... blonde woman... Eva, is always hanging around her room. I was waiting for just the right time to..."

Interrupting him before he could finish, Dalton gritted out, "Find out who she is, and then get her out of the way. I don't care how. Just do it. And call Susan. Tell her to ready one of my apartments for a new employee on standby. I'm sending a potentially useful asset to the States on the next flight out. I want you to keep a close watch on her. She could be of some use to me later on. She is weak-minded and easily controlled. Keep Susan informed at all times, and tell her not to talk to anyone."

The man answered him confidently. "Yes, sir. I will just as soon as I end this call."

"Very good. And don't disappoint me again." Dalton

ended the call and nodded to his driver. "I'm ready." The impressively dressed man swiftly got out of the driver's side and opened the back door. Stepping out, Dalton straightened his pants and buttoned the jacket of his tailored suit. He looked around at his new surroundings. Scrunching his nose in disgust, Dalton sneered his extreme dislike of the place.

Everything smelled damp, mossy, and fishy. He hated it. The door to the house opened before they even made it to the walkway. Though too skinny for his preference, the blonde drank him in with appreciation. She was obviously excited about his worth in dollar signs. So… she was one of *those* women. He could use that to his advantage.

Her smile grew wider, and she gave a shy wave as he approached. "Well, hello there, boys. Come, bring yourselves inside. We have a lot to discuss."

Dalton turned to his driver. "Wait in the car until I'm finished here." He turned his back, dismissing him. The bleached-blonde was obviously surprised by his curt dismissal of the man. She had a moment's pause, seemingly apprehensive about inviting Dalton, a complete stranger and foreigner, into her home. She hesitated by the open doorway, but Dalton pushed forward.

He bumped her out of the way, hard, causing her to stumble back into the house. "It's too late to change your mind now, princess. I've already flown out here. The decision has been made." He shoved her aside like he owned the place. Dalton walked through the front room and down the hall. Not knowing what else to do in the presence of this powerfully imposing man, Shannon hustled after him. She kept her distance, though, staying a few steps behind him. She was frightened and unsure what would happen next. Dalton made his way to her tiny kitchen.

"Shitty place you've got here! No wonder you want out of here so bad." The blonde-in-a-box glowered at him, her brows dipping low giving away her growing anger. This only egged him on even more. "Oh, did I offend you, Shannon? If you love it here so much, I'll just be on my way. I'm sure there is someone else who could reap the benefits of my wealthy offer…"

Biting her lip, she reached out to him. "No, wait. I… I do want to go to the States. It is a once in a lifetime opportunity for me. It's just your lack of manners that raises my anger so. I don't like the way you speak to me." She finished her predictable speech, lifting her head in pride. Dalton's lip curled over his white teeth in an eerie grin. He would enjoy putting her in her place.

Motioning to the chair at the kitchenette table, he barked out at her, "Sit! Now, Shannon, you *will* tell me everything you know about Grady's Pub—all the people who frequent it, and the times they usually come and go. That includes your ex."

Shannon jumped out of her chair, pacing back and forth in her kitchen and continued to chew her lip nervously. This sounded extremely wrong to her. "Why do you want to know about him? I thought you just wanted information about that bitch he's with... Ellora."

Dalton had to stop himself from striking this despicable woman across her mouth. His face turned crimson with rage as he forced himself to hold back the urge to hurt her. Who does this woman think she is? How dare she talk about his dark beauty in such a way. She doesn't even hold a candle to her magnificence.

He forced his next words out through tightly gritted teeth. "Don't you EVER talk about her in that manner again." Shannon jumped at his threatening tone. "Do. You. Understand? What I want and why is not your concern, is it?" His manic expression and sinister sneer startled her, and she shook her head frantically, not wanting to anger him any further.

His tone dropped. Dalton pointed a finger at her accusingly. "I'll take you back to the States so you can start the new life you've always dreamed of, in exchange for any information I need to know. Are you saying you want to back out?"

Shannon's eyes grew wide, afraid she was about to lose out on the opportunity offered to her over the phone. An opportunity of a lifetime. Dalton watched semi-amused as she finally decided to show him just how much she really wanted the deal.

She tried her best to pull off a runway model strut

across the room toward him. Flipping her hair over her shoulder, the overly made up blonde winked at him flirtatiously, pointing to the other chair in the small kitchen. "Sit down. I'll show you how much I want this opportunity and how much I appreciate you giving it to me."

The self-righteous, dominant, master manipulator did not like being told what to do. He despised being questioned. If she only knew she already had two strikes against her, she wouldn't dare toy with him like she was trying to do.

"Anything, huh? You think you've got what it takes to handle a man of my caliber?" Shannon nodded, eyeing him up and down. This chick actually thought she had a chance with a man of Dalton's status. Yeah, right. She was beneath him. She was trash. Nothing and no one compared to Ellora.

Shannon gasped out in shock when this neatly put together man lunged out unexpectedly and grabbed her by the back of her head, pulling on her hair. It tangled in his clenched fist as he dragged her across the room and over to her chair.

"Prove it to me. Right now." Dalton forced her down on her knees. She cried out in fright as he unzipped his tailored pants. The vile man yanked her head back all the way so she could see his face, and hissed, "Go ahead. Show me what you've got. You were so eager a few minutes ago. This is what you want, right?"

Shannon's terrified eyes and shaking hesitation

pleased the evil man. A cruel smile spread across his merciless face. "I didn't think so!" Dalton pushed her head roughly aside and zipped up his pants. "Don't put all your cards on the table if you're not willing to follow through and play them."

She crawled to the corner, as far away from him as possible, and sobbed silently. What did she get herself into? She should've paid attention to the warning bells that sounded off inside her head at his 'too good to be true' offer.

Dalton slowly strode over to where she sat trembling. Frightened as to what he might do to her next, she shook violently at his approach. "Oh, don't worry. I wouldn't touch you if you offered yourself up on a platinum platter. You are not my type." He looked down on her with complete disdain. "The moment you accepted my offer... that was it. Your choices and decisions are out of your hands now. The deal is set in stone."

The terrified girl shook her head in disbelief. How had she gotten into this mess? She didn't want to tell him anything about Behr. But she also didn't want to get hurt, or pass up a ticket out of there. Dalton gritted his teeth and clenched his fists as his anger and frustration grew from her lack of cooperation. His patience was teetering on the edge. If she made one more stupid decision, he would strike her.

"I'm losing my patience with you, Shannon. You don't want a man like me as your enemy. With a snap of my fingers, I could have you shipped off to one of many human trafficking rings and sell you to the highest bidder. It would be an easy enough task. No one would go looking for someone like you. Everyone here knows how badly you want to leave. And that, my dear, is the kindest option awaiting you. I could think of far more twisted scenarios, where I can have your family involved as well. Is that what you want?"

"No! No, please. I will cooperate. I'm... I'm sorry, Dalton. Sir." Ashamed and still in a state of shock, she stood on shaky legs.

Dalton motioned his hand over to the empty seat. "Tell me, Shannon. Tell me all you know. How can I get close to her?"

Shannon's voice trembled as she searched her scared and incoherent thoughts, trying to think of a way he could get close to her undetected. His anger intensified as he waited impatiently at her silence. Without thinking, Shannon blurted out, "She lives on the second floor flat at Grady's. But there is an unused third floor flat. Not many know, but you can gain access to it from outside. There is an old rusted out fire escape that is covered in ivy, as it's gone unused for decades. No one goes up there."

Dalton snaked his thin lips over her forehead, placing a revolting kiss.

"Good girl."

"Hey, Behr. So, tell me how it feels to be back on the water." Ellora balanced her cell in between her shoulder and ear while sanding down the freshly spackled sheetrock. The place already looked one-hundred percent better after she hung them on all the walls.

"Aye, it's a beautiful day for it, that's for sure. I was just checkin' in to see if you're a'right and if you need me for anythin', love."

Ellora decided she'd tease him a little bit. He'd been calling every hour asking her the same questions. "There is something I need from you, Behr..." Dropping her voice a few seductive octaves, she said in a husky tone, "But, it has nothing to do with work... and everything to do with being alone with you."

Ellora held in her laugh when he choked, stammering and sputtering on the other line. She couldn't hold it in any longer and finally let her laugh go, snorting like a pig. "Ha! That's what happens when you ask the same question for the hundredth time in a row... Ninety-nine times is my limit, Behr. You're all out."

Behr's roaring laughter crackled through the speakers on her phone as the bass in his voice thundered on the other line. "Ah, you lil' she-devil. You'll pay for that. Nearly killed me, ya did. I'm docking now at the terminal. Didja want to go to Grady's for a bite? I could meet you there and walk you down, love."

Ellora beamed as she heard him exiting the busy

terminal. Behr would go out of his way for her, without exception, even if it didn't make sense. Always the thoughtful gentleman. "No, that's okay. I'll meet you at Grady's. It's half-way for the both of us."

Behr sighed in resignation. "I'd really rather walk with my girl on my arm down there. But, I know how stubborn you are." He chuckled lightly, changing the subject. "So how's my favorite handy woman today?"

Smiling from ear to ear, the busy girl stopped what she was doing to sit down. "I'm doing all right, just sanding down the sheetrock on the walls. I should be ready to paint in a week. The custom windows I ordered will be here the day after tomorrow. Thank God! I'll finally be able to take the plywood off the windows." Ellora hesitated for a moment. "It gets super creepy in here sometimes."

"What do you mean, sweetheart? Would you like me to walk through the place again?" After her attack, Behr had become adamant about checking every single room before Ellora ever stepped foot in it... Even at Grady's. He always walked in her little apartment and made sure it was safe before he left her side for the night. His fear and touching concern was giving him a major case of OCD. It pulled at her heart strings.

"No. It's just... I don't know. I feel like I'm being watched or something. I get this sinking feeling, like I'm not alone in here. Maybe this old building is haunted or something?" Ellora forced out a laugh, feeling silly for saying it out loud.

"Maybe it's your ma and da watching over you," Behr suggested, trying to ease her nerves.

"No, it's a completely different feeling I get. It makes my stomach sick. Sometimes, it reminds me of… of the time I walked into a room in my father's house and *he* was there."

Ellora didn't get a chance to finish her sentence. Behr's voice dropped in seriousness. It sounded like he was her very own warrior. "I'm coming!" Before Ellora could tell him it was just a stupid feeling, that she'd probably just imagined it, and she'd meet him at Grady's, he hung up the phone. Checking the time on her cell, Ellora gave him five minutes before he burst through the door like a beast on a mission.

She dropped what she was doing and hurried to the door. *Oh shit. My bags.* Ellora cursed, turning back to grab her stuff. Bending down, she reached out to snatch up her backpack and tool belt, when she froze on the spot. The whole world shifted on its axis. A slight breeze wafted at her back, and the hairs on the back of her neck stood in warning. Icy chills trickled down her spine, because there were no windows or doors open for this to be possible. A dark figure moved out of the corner of her eye.

She wasn't crazy, she told herself over and over. She may have been hyperaware, but she'd seen it! She knew she did. All the blood drained from her face as she got up enough nerve and slowly turned around. With dilated eyes, her adrenaline flooded her system. A cold sweat broke out all over, causing her shirt to stick to her skin.

"Don't freeze up this time, Lor... Go!" She emboldened herself. Dropping the bags, Ellora sprinted toward the door. She flung it open harder than necessary. Bursting through it, she was momentarily blinded when the bright sun shone on her face, and then she crashed into a wall of hard steel.

Behr. Oh, thank God.

Tears dripped down her paling face. Now that she was wrapped securely in his strong, protective arms, Ellora blushed. Her reaction seemed extremely foolish now.

Obviously, she must've imagined the whole thing. After all, she was still skittish inside that building after her last attack, and must've psyched herself out talking about ghosts with Behr. It was just her imagination... Right?

"Ellora! What happened? Are you a'right? What's going on?" He flooded her with questions and only stopped when his green-eyed beauty spoke up.

"Nothing. It's... I'm okay. I think I just got scared, that's all. I've been cooped up in that dark warehouse for far too long. I think I must've just been hallucinating." A shaky laugh came out nervously, not convincing him in the least, given the circumstances. A few more fat tears rolled down her dampened cheeks.

She was tired and overworked. The hours of hard labor and lack of rest left her suspicious and paranoid. She was making herself crazy. Now would be a good time for a break. Behr softly shushed her as he held her tighter to him.

"What is it you thought you saw, love?" he asked, kissing the top of her dusty head.

"I don't know. I thought I saw a dark figure right behind me out of the corner of my eye. It was probably just the sinking feeling in my gut again, really." Her giant protector rubbed her back in soothing circles, shaking his head in disagreement.

"No. You should always trust your gut instincts, love. They are a God given gift, an internal warning system. It is what has kept you alive in the past. Don't second guess it, and don't second guess yourself. C'mon, Lor, let's get something to eat, yeah? Gavin and I will head back here later to do a thorough walk through, to double check the place."

"Okay." Ellora's voice came out sounding very fragile and small to her own ears.

It was all she could say. An eerie, horrid, nausea churned in warning deep in the pit of her stomach. She wasn't sure what brought on such an intense reaction, but she definitely didn't want to be alone in there anymore.

Looking back at the abandoned warehouse one more time, Ellora was led away by Behr, tucked safely into his side. She could've sworn she caught sight of a shadow by the cracked glass in the window of the busted door. After forcefully blinking a few times, she looked again… and the shadow was gone. It was probably just the glare of the sun playing tricks on her… she hoped.

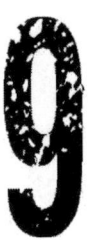

roup session ended, and Giddeon waited patiently in the hallway for Eva, watching the other members shuffle out the door. He refused to share anything this week, and he could tell she was royally pissed at him. It's not that he was trying to be difficult; he just couldn't bring himself to say anything. The idea of letting a bunch of strangers into his twisted mind, actually telling his story out loud while they eyeballed him, made everything too... *real*.

The smell of her delicate perfume made it out into the hallway before his Angel did. Walking through the threshold, Eva jumped at the sight of Giddeon. "Holy shit! You scared the crap outta me." Her outburst generated a smile from him. His Angel had such a dirty mouth. He looked down at her tempting bow-shaped lips. Eva noticed the gesture, narrowed her eyes, and pursed her lips. "What is it, Giddeon?"

Her agitation took him aback. "I'm sorry, Angel. I didn't mean to scare you."

Eva watched as he reached out and absentmindedly tucked a stray hair behind her ear, distracting her from her bad mood.

"Can we have dinner tonight? Let me take you to dinner." Giddeon was just as shocked as she looked, left staring in disbelief as the off-topic and very random sentence left his mouth. It wasn't what Giddeon wanted to say at all, but once uttered, he had to own it.

Eva snatched the hair he just tucked away and aggressively untucked it. Chuckling, he shook his head at her defiance. "What? Like on a date? Hell no! Giddeon, I'm your group leader! And... and... you're a mess. I mean no offense... I'm not judging. I've been where you are."

Her quick refusal stung a little. "I doubt it," he mumbled under his breath.

Eva continued without pause, "Open up. Use the group to get yourself right, okay?" Giddeon thought about what she said for a minute, but once again, his mouth jumped the gun. "How about lunch? A feisty girl like you has got to have a good healthy appetite on her."

His golden Angel lifted an amused brow and smirked at him. "You just don't quit, do you? I should give you a break because you're new, but I know you could do better if you actually tried. Make an effort in group... for me, okay? Otherwise, you'll make me look bad in there, all right." She winked at him and crossed her arms over her chest. This action pushed her cleavage up in a tantalizing fashion.

Completely mesmerized, Giddeon would've done anything she'd asked him to do. "How about if you have coffee with me, and I'll tell you a story from my past. C'mon... coffee is harmless, right?"

Giddeon could've sworn she whispered back, "You're anything but harmless."

They stood staring at each other for a countless amount of time. Giddeon could almost see the wheels turning as she thought about his offer, and wished he could climb inside of that beautiful head of hers to see what her answer would be.

Doubt was working its way into Giddeon's mind during her extended silence, and just when he thought she was going to reject him again, Eva placed her hands on her hips in a self-assured stance and relented. "Okay. One coffee for one confession. You've got yourself a deal."

Shit. He actually told her he'd give her a confession, didn't he? He thought he said that in his head. Guess not. Grabbing his cold, marked-up arm, Eva urged him down the hall before he could back out of the deal. "C'mon, I'll take you to my favorite place. Call the detective and let him know we moved our 'meeting'," she used air quotes when saying it, "across the street so he doesn't flip out, okay?" Giddeon's heart raced when she rubbed her delicate hands over his roughened forearms.

They walked the short distance to The Fix, a little coffee shop across the street. Eva oooed and aaahed as she closed her eyes, breathing in the intoxicating aroma of foreign dark-roast coffee beans. "What's your poison,

Angel?" She ordered a mocha something or other with whipped cream and chocolate syrup drizzled on top.

"Oh, yeah! That's what I needed. Come to mama." Giddeon could've sworn a whooshing noise followed when Eva snatched the coffee cup into her greedy hands. He couldn't help but smile at the adorable noises she was making while sipping the decadent caffeine fix.

"That coffee must be something else."

Eva just mumbled in agreement, "Mmm hmm."

"Do you make those same noises in bed, Angel? Or is that just a special treat that I got to witness?"

She scoffed, throwing him a murderous glare for his question. "Wouldn't you like to know?"

"She's a feisty one today." The otherwise serious man curled his fingers, mimicking a hissing cat, and finally after all her snarkiness, Giddeon was rewarded with a smile. They walked to the back of the shop and settled into a tiny booth for two next to the windows.

At long last, he finally had her alone, in a quiet, intimate surrounding. Her tongue darted out to capture a runaway drop of the exquisite coffee. The light-haired beauty eyed him suspiciously when she caught him gazing over her, longing to sample those plump lips. "So, mystery man, what's your story?"

Dragging his eyes away from the temptation of her wetted lips, the dark man met her blue eyes with his black ones. "What is it you want to know about me, counsellor?"

Swirling her coffee, deep in thought, his group leader thoroughly searched over his face, then lowered her eyes. "Hmmm…"

Looking at her expressive face, Giddeon could see the moment Eva decided on a question.

Leaning across the tiny table, Eva reached out her hand and brushed her fingers with a feather-light touch along his most dreadfully jagged scar. The scar tissue along his neck was full of sensitive nerves. Obviously, no one had ever touched him there. His usually numb body tingled with delight at her strangely erotic touch. He hissed out a breath through his clenched teeth, and his fists tightened, trying to refrain from grabbing her and pulling her into his cut up arms.

The brave girl only hesitated for a second at his reaction. When he made no move to stop her, she continued. Her fingers danced back and forth along this shameful reminder of his tragic past that he couldn't escape from.

"How did you get this scar, Giddeon?"

He grasped her arm, carefully pulling it away. He didn't let go, just ran his hand softly down her tiny forearm. When he reached her hand, his calloused fingers attentively drew imaginary circles on her palm, nodding his head. "Yeah. I can give you that story. Don't expect an easy answer. You're not going to like it, and you'll like me even less than you do now."

Strong-willed, Eva took hold of the hand playing with

hers and enveloped hers around it with a supportive touch. "I would never judge you. Never."

When Giddeon shook his head in disagreement, Eva stopped the motion by cupping his face.

"We all have terrible pasts. Our character is built and strengthened by how we move past our tragedies. You have to push against the darkness that tries to drag you back under. People like us have to fight our way to happiness, but you have to really want it. What matters, Giddeon, is the here and now. Grab your chance at a new life and don't let go. I will be here to help you as best as I can. Trust in me enough to let me in. But, in the end, only you can make the transition and change. Good or bad, I'll be here if you need me."

Another fissure split down the wall protecting his heart. His chest caved from the emptiness that he had been numb to for so many years. The weight of this new sensation crushed his heart. The pain was just too real. Broken, he hung his head in shame. He couldn't look at her while he told this story. Eva softly rubbed his stubble-roughened cheeks with her thumbs in soothing circles. "I'm right here, Giddeon. No matter what you tell me, I will be right here. I'm not going anywhere."

After taking in a steadying breath, he began his story. "Most kids at the age of six are afraid of the dark, spiders, clowns... I don't know normal shit like that. Not me. My childhood fears were different. When I was placed in the first of many foster homes, the horror of what happened to me was still very raw. I'd wake every night, all night long, screaming. It really freaked my foster parents out. Every time my eyes closed, I was haunted by the sounds of my mother's screams as they gutted her, ripping her wide open. The undeniable realization that I just stood there, frozen, unable to move or lift a finger to help, tore me apart with guilt.

"My sanity was slowly slipping away from me, just like the life from their eyes. The struggle to forget what I witnessed was an everyday battle, but the horror was always right there behind my eyes, like a monster banging down the door that I desperately tried to keep closed. I was such a coward. I wasn't strong enough to fight away my fears, and I definitely didn't know how to deal with them. People kept telling me that I'd still feel my parents' spirits with me, feel them in here." Giddeon pointed to his heart and tapped on his chest.

Eva sat back, listening to the heart wrenching nightmare Giddeon spewed out, trying with all her strength to listen to every word and not interrupt. It proved to be extremely difficult. All she wanted to do was gather the broken man into the safety of her arms and never let go. Tears tried to force their way out, burning her eyes as she fought to hold them back.

Blowing out a withered breath, Giddeon continued. "But, all I could feel was despair in my heart. Those wounds never lessened over time. They never healed. My foster parents never once sat by my bed with me during my tough nights, never wiped away my tears, or held me tight to them. They never once comforted me through my terrifying night terrors. They didn't care about me. They just wanted their government issued check. Caring about me had been my parents' job. I finally had to convince myself that they were really gone and that they were never coming back for me. I was truly alone in the world. I had turned emotionally void... cold."

Giddeon ran his hands through his hair, then fisting a handful of it, he pulled tight with frustration. "I was so tired of just existing. I was numb to everything else around me. I decided at seven years old, on the one-year anniversary of their murder, that I didn't want to be here anymore. I wanted to end my never ending suffering... I wanted to die. That thought was the only thing that had me excited in a very long time. I would meet up with my parents in heaven, where I would finally get to hold them tight again. My mom would kiss me all over my face. My dad would lift me up off the ground, hug me tight to him, and squeeze, just like he used to do.

"That wonderful thought, paired with the overwhelming feeling of loneliness, was so powerful that I didn't even hesitate. I grabbed the dagger I'd kept hidden in the springs of my bed and pressed as hard as I could, dragging it across my throat. I remember being shocked at first, at the sight of my own blood spraying out and splattering everywhere. Then, I just remember feeling euphoric. The pain made me feel things again. It relaxed me.

"I laid on my bed, bleeding out and waiting for death to claim me. I closed my eyes, picturing their happy faces as they greeted me to my everlasting home. I'd be reunited with them forever. Nothing would ever separate us again.

"My dreams were crushed when my foster parents walked into my room with the CPS representative for their monthly visit. They were still ordered to check up on me. They packed me up and sent me to a mental health hospital for emotionally traumatized kids. I was there for a long time. I despised it there and learned fairly quickly to fake 'normal' pretty well.

"I think I was thirteen when they finally let me out. I had become a very angry teen with an exceptionally large chip on my shoulder. They shipped me off to the next foster nightmare then." His voice faded away to an almost inaudible whisper as he finished his story. Finally lifting his head, he avoided looking into Eva's eyes, gazing instead out the window. Carefree people walked the sidewalks, hustling back to their jobs from their lunch breaks. His idle mind wondered if his parents would even recognize him now if they saw him.

They didn't even know each other anymore. They were virtually strangers. Giddeon was not even close to the boy they knew and loved. He guessed it didn't matter anyway; it's not like he'd ever be allowed up there with them. Not after all he'd done, and not when he could feel the Devil pulling him down into the darkness with him.

The broken man continued to look outside, avoiding the eyes of the woman who sat listening. He didn't have the heart to look and see what she was feeling, or see what she might've thought about him. He couldn't handle it at that moment. His heart was ripped wide open, raw and bleeding, right there in front of her. His story had left him vulnerable, and he hated that helpless feeling. Giddeon had to focus hard on rebuilding the walls around his breaking heart, back up to where they used to be.

"Oh, Giddeon," his Angel whispered, her heart aching for him. He could hear it in the sound of her voice. She got up from her chair and walked around behind the emotionally broken man. Leaning down, she draped her arms around him. Eva's hand rested on top of his. He could've sat like that forever. Her embrace was strong, caring, and somewhat familiar.

It wasn't a pitying embrace, but supportive, understanding. If he wasn't mistaken, Eva genuinely cared about him.

No. He couldn't let himself think about that. It'd give him hope. No one had ever cared about him besides his parents. Who could possibly care for a fucked up, piece of shit like him anyways? Giddeon was nothing but a twisted, sick coward.

Eva lowered her head beside his ear and nuzzled against his neck. As if reading his mind, she declared, "Oh, Giddeon, you are worth so much more than you believe." She squeezed him tighter. "You deserve this. You deserve to be cared for. Every human being needs that. You should allow yourself to be loved. You've been through enough already. Everything has been taken away from you. It's okay to be a little selfish. Take a breath and just live your life. Your parents would want that for you."

Irritation rose up to the surface. *She doesn't know a fucking thing about what they'd want.* Grabbing her arm, Giddeon yanked her around to face him. He wanted to tell her as much. Eva took the angry man off guard when she flung her leg over his lap and straddled him. This unexpected action stunned him. She was always doing this—shocking him, catching him off guard, and challenging him outside of his comfort zone.

Gone were any thoughts of anger or despair. The once dangerous hit-man, in that moment, thought of nothing else besides this golden Angel sitting in his lap. Cupping his face in her hands, she not so gently forced his head up to meet her eyes. Leaning her forehead against his, she answered Giddeon's unspoken thoughts. "I do know, all too well. And I am right. Try to prove me otherwise."

The heavy weight of her genuine concern opened his eyes, but Giddeon couldn't let himself fall for her. She deserved so much better than the shell of a man she was gazing at. He wouldn't let this happen. Eva's face hardened when she watched his demeanor close itself off from her. "Don't. Don't do this." Her voice sounded foreign as the words came out harshly in warning.

Giddeon lifted her easily off of his lap and carefully placed her back down on his seat. "Sorry, Angel. Some people can't be saved." But the stubborn woman shook her head in disagreement. Not to be swayed, Giddeon finished before she could start. "Some people just aren't worth it. I hope you enjoy your coffee." Turning on his heel, Giddeon aimed for the front of the shop and his exit out. He made it about a dozen steps or so before she caught up to him. This stubborn woman never gave up.

"Are you... am I going to see you in group next week, Giddeon?"

For some reason, his chest ached at the sound of her voice as she whispered his name. The way it rolled off her tongue in that way sounded intimate.

His voice softened as well. "I don't know. Dominick and I are following some leads that he's been working on." When she gave him a look that pleaded with him to stay with her, he clenched his fists in frustration.

He had to stay focused. She had distracted him enough. Giddeon had to remember his end goal. Justice for his slain parents. And revenge. He would have both. He promised them both... and he promised himself. He couldn't let this girl get in the way of that. "I won't have time to think about anything else," he said in a tone harsher than necessary. A brief look of disappointment showed on her face. It must've been because he was her new subject to fix, because it couldn't be that she actually cared about him.

"Giddeon..." Before he had a chance to think, react, or respond, Eva placed a soft lingering kiss on his stiff lips, jolting him out of his thoughts. She was out the door before he could even blink an eye. He had been left standing there, staring after her. Another crack inside his chest broke the once impenetrable wall that kept him numb and unfeeling. Bulldozing her way into his heart, no matter how hard he tried to stop it from happening, she was getting inside. Eva was leaving her mark. The once cold organ was flooded by warm electrical currents that roused his body from its long petrified state.

Giddeon would be lying to himself if he thought for one moment that he wouldn't be thinking about her while he was gone. Because of that kiss, he wouldn't be able to think of anything else. With one soft touch from her exquisite lips, she had dashed all of his plans to stay focused on his parents.

Every time he tried to refocus his mind on their revenge, her sweet face rushed into his consciousness, and everything else would fall away. Just look at him... He was still standing in the middle of a busy coffee shop, frozen to the spot. He could think of nothing else but her.

Finally, when he realized people were trying to walk

in or out without disturbing him, his brain caught up with the rest of him and told his feet to start moving. His overpowering presence gave him a wide berth of space. They didn't dare ask him to move out of the way. "All right, Giddeon," he mumbled to himself, clapping his hands to wake himself up. "Let's get your pansy ass back to work."

Giddeon walked out of the shop while dialing Dominick's number. "C'mon, Detective, are we going to start working here or what? Let's do this."

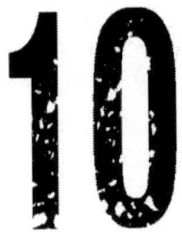

ominick and Giddeon stormed the office in Dalton's high-rise. The detective ordered his unusual partner to hang back, knowing that Giddeon's presence tended to frighten others, and he didn't want their next possible witness to clam up. So, Dominick decided to use the 'Detective approach', hoping to convince Susan, Dalton's personal assistant, to talk. She worked side-by-side with the man himself for years. He ran everything by her. She had to know his whereabouts.

Dominick used an old trick that usually worked well for him, from when he was back on the beat. He'd threaten her with evidence that they had in their possession, which, of course, they didn't. Dominick was hoping that putting fear of prosecution under obstruction and aiding and abetting charges would be enough to have Susan spill her guts.

Giddeon sat crouching outside the door, listening. The detective tried interrogating the stubborn, tight-lipped girl for a few more minutes, to no avail. She wasn't budging. The once dangerous hit-man knew she wouldn't dare talk… not to Dominick, anyway. Dalton retained and controlled his employees' allegiances by having something very important to that person under his thumb. That precious 'something' was different to each person, but each feared losing.

Susan feared Dalton so much, she ended up being his most reliable asset. After all, she had the most to lose. Giddeon knew this about her. They had come to be employed by Dalton around the same time several years ago. She had been easily controlled by Dalton right off the bat.

Losing all patience, Giddeon charged through the door and into the office. Susan paled at the sight of the monster standing before her. He was the only other man in the world she feared as much as, if not more than, Dalton himself. Susan had been present in several instances of her boss's version of 'negotiations'. The frightened young girl witnessed first-hand the monster Giddeon truly was. She was the only person to see the beast when he was unleashed from inside of him and still be alive afterward.

The neatly dressed girl quaked under the heavy weight of Giddeon's evil glare as he stalked toward them. Dalton was clearly not around to keep her safe from him— not very wise on his part. His devious mentality took over; Giddeon would use her fear to get what he wanted out of her.

With purpose in his steps, he stormed across the office, past Dominick, aiming straight for Susan. His cold, dark eyes trained solely on hers. The girl's face turned ashen gray as all the blood drained from her face. The strength had left her body while the monster assaulted her with nothing more than the power of his lethal intent. The same way he looked on all his unfortunate victims.

Clutching the desk in front of her, Susan tried to steady herself as her whole body shook. She'd always been uncontrollably petrified of this immoral monster. He starred in her nightmares. Still holding the secretary prisoner with his entrancing black eyes, Giddeon growled out at the equally shocked detective, "Get out! Give me the room. And no matter what you hear... Do. Not. Come. In."

The already petrified girl's eyes widened. Panicking, she looked to the detective with pleading eyes. Shaking her head back and forth, her fear crippled her ability to speak. Dominick's natural instincts were to serve and protect. It showed in his hesitation to leave. The marked man whipped his head around to his partner. Already dangerously close to the edge, Giddeon bellowed out when he didn't move fast enough, "Get the fuck out of here, Detective! This is what I do."

Dominick gave him a warning glare of his own that said, 'better not hurt her'. Hesitantly, he forced his feet to move out of the office. The sound of the heavy mahogany door clicked closed, sealing the girl's fate as she was left alone with a monster. The sound echoed around the room, giving it a sense of finality. Giddeon knew that she would feel it in the depth of her bones.

Without pause or warning, the murderer she'd feared

all these years charged at her with startling speed. The only sound that made it out of her petrified form was a screeching cry. Backing away from the expansive desk, she tripped several times on shaky legs. A weak attempt on her part at putting distance between them.

The sinister man jumped the desk all too easily, with the poise of an Olympic hurdler. Once over, he threw the heavily carved captain's chair out of his way. With nowhere else to go, Susan flattened herself against Dalton's massive bookshelf. Tears made a trail down her powdered cheeks.

Giddeon caged her like a hungry beast trapping its prey. He knew Dalton kept her loyal by using his favorite method: fear and leverage. Susan had a mother in a nursing home who needed round the clock care, and a little brother in a special needs school—both of which were fully funded by Dalton. She had a lot to lose… And they both knew it.

"Who did Dalton use to put that woman in the hospital? The one who's now in a coma? Who is he using now that I'm out of the picture?" His anger grew after each question remained unanswered. His voice rose higher and higher. The girl cringed as he bellowed out one question after another. When her mouth opened and nothing came out, Giddeon snapped.

Grabbing her neck, the cold-blooded man applied pressure, squeezing callously. "Tell me! Or, so help me God, I'll tear them into pieces that you'll never find."

She gurgled inaudibly, so he loosened his grip a

fraction. "They are both the same man... the man he used before you. Let me go and I'll get all I have on him... from over there." She pointed in the general direction of the desk. "But, he isn't one who can be found unless he wants to be. Without so much as a phone call from Dalton, he knew you were caught somehow. He just showed up out of the blue. He knew everything already, and just like you, this man truly enjoys what he does."

Giddeon hated the man already. He immediately wanted to take him on. It sounded like it'd be a challenging fight.

Grabbing the choking girl by the hair, he dragged her over to the desk. "Get it! Quickly!" Susan knocked over several items because of her trembling hands, and the rest of her body shook uncontrollably as she fought to keep herself upright. She reached out to a cigar keepsake box on his desk and pulled out a key from its false bottom. She opened it slowly, and Giddeon found himself leaning forward to see what was inside.

There were dozens of pictures of Ellora inside.

"Sick fuck!" He snatched the pictures out of the box and flipped through. Each one was creepier than the last. There were several of Ellora working on the job here at a pretty young age. There were more of her loading groceries into a cart. The last one looked like it was taken outside a window, looking in. The dark-haired girl was sprawled across the carpet in her room with papers around her...

homework possibly.

This guy had fucking problems. He let himself wallow in guilt for the briefest of moments for what he'd done to her, for what he'd almost followed through with. He almost dragged that poor girl back to this crazy dipshit. He didn't want to think about what might've happened to her if he'd succeeded. A moment of realization came to him. Eva had said that the more you confess your sins out loud, and listen in on the problems of others, your mind starts to recognize the addictive habit, and you could stop yourself from continuing the pattern.

Giddeon didn't want to hurt Susan, not like he used to enjoy hurting people. That level of cruelty was now reserved for Dalton... and, of course, his parents' killers. Even though Susan stood in his way of getting what he needed, and he'd still do anything to get it, Giddeon didn't want to hurt her. She, too, was a victim of Dalton's greed, manipulations, and unlimited connections. Just like everyone else, she was stuck in his web and couldn't find her way out. Susan did what she was forced to do in order to survive under his punishing rule.

Grasping the keys with unsteady hands, Susan walked over to an industrial-sized filing cabinet with a keyed lock. Jackpot! It took her well over ten minutes to find the right file and hand it to him. The dark man took hold of her chin as gently as he was able, which wasn't that gentle at all as anger still coursed through his veins. He forced her head up to meet his eyes. "You understand why I'm doing this, don't you?"

The frightened girl shook her head 'no.'

"He blackmails and manipulates us all. He has ruined countless lives, and uses people like us to do all the heavy lifting for him. No more! This all ends. Soon. I promise." She nodded just to pacify him. He let her go and stalked toward the door. "If I were you... I'd pull all the files on those who've mysteriously gone missing under his employment, then get ready for a career change, sweetheart. The detective will be back to pick them up when you least expect him, so have them ready."

"Yes... Yes, Giddeon. I will," she stuttered, still in utter shock by his threatening presence and having her whole world dragged down around her. She may not know it yet, but Giddeon was doing her a solid favor. His old self wouldn't have given her a chance; he would've just choked the life out of her so she couldn't tell anyone of his plans, and walked away.

Which reminded him... Giddeon turned on his heel and quickly launched himself at her once more. "I swear, Susan, if you tell Dalton anything, or let on about what's been done... I will torture your little brother, force him to watch me kill his mother, before I force you to watch me kill him. Your death will give me endless hours of fun as I drag it out. Maybe a few days. Weeks. Not a word uttered. Do. You. Understand?" Giddeon had no intention of following through with this threat, but he wanted to make sure Susan wouldn't stray from their plan.

She was now a blubbering mess after hearing his malicious threat. Her tears streamed down her face and neck like a running faucet. "Yes. Yes, I will do whatever you want. Just, please… Don't hurt them. I won't say anything."

"Good girl." Giddeon walked out the door, meeting a worried Dominick in the hallway. Slapping him on the shoulder, he handed him the file and walked right past him. "All right, Detective, you're up. Start detecting."

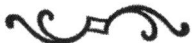

Behr looked over as the movie came to an end. The glow of the flat screen softly cast rosy shadows across Ellora's porcelain face. She was still very shaken up by what she thought she saw earlier, and what she sensed deep down in her gut. It took several hours to help calm her nerves. Curling up beside her in bed, watching a b-rated romantic comedy did the trick.

Leaning in, he cherished the sight of his love as she yawned long and hard, gesturing her need for sleep. He couldn't explain why, but he was compelled to remain by her side. The thought of abandoning her for the night to sleep in his own bed had a knot twisting in his gut; it was overwhelmingly wrong. After her expressed fears over the phone, and the way she leapt into his arms at the warehouse, a sinking feeling dwelled deep inside him. Behr never wanted to leave her there all alone to begin with, but didn't want her to think he was suffocating her. This time, it was different.

After watching Giddeon attack her in that very same building, he'd had to fight the need to stay by her side every waking moment from that day forward. Whenever she was frightened, his protective instincts took over. In fact, the only time he ever felt out of control was when she wasn't by his side. He squeezed her soft, petite body in the protective cage of his strong arms. Softly laying kiss after kiss on her neck, he thought about how he would risk his life again and again to keep her safe.

Half-heartedly, Behr untangled their limbs. His plan was to tuck her in, make sure all was well, and leave, just like every other evening. But, he longed for just one night, just one night to sleep soundly wrapped in each other's arms. It would probably upset her if he asked, because he knew she wasn't ready. By the way Ellora was settling impossibly closer into his arms, however, he guessed she wanted him to be close to her just as much. Deciding against it, Behr reluctantly placed a soft kiss on her adorable pouty lips. "Good night, my love. I'll let you get some sleep. See you t'morrow morn... I love you."

Ellora quickly stopped him before he got up. "No. I want you to stay with me."

Behr gazed at her for a moment, gauging her response.

"If at any time t' night, my being 'ere makes you uncomfortable..."

"I need you. Please, don't go." Her pleading was his undoing. There was nothing in this world he wanted more.

"Aye, your wish is my command, love. Let me remove my shoes and ready myself for bed then, a'right?"

Ellora couldn't help but watch the impressive man as he rose from the bed that they'd been tangled up in moments ago. The cold absence he left behind affected her the instant he left her side. An overwhelming ache spread throughout her trembling body as she waited, needing to feel his arms wrap around her once again. Behr turned, facing her as he kicked off his shoes and removed his socks. The soft light from the lamp posts on the pier outside trickled through the window, illuminating beautifully all around him.

Behr raised once more, immense and imposing, his keen eyes exploring the exquisite beauty that lay sprawled out... waiting for him. He was the most fortunate man on earth that she'd stumbled into his life and chose him. Clutching a fistful of fabric, Behr pulled his shirt up over his head and tossed it aside. When his eyes found hers, he was astonished when longing burned hot and bright in Ellora's eyes as she gazed up at him in the most intimately vulnerable way. That expression nearly pushed him over the edge and had his head spinning. He wanted her in the worst way.

Ellora's temperature rose higher, burning her slowly from the inside out as she beheld the glow of the lights outside splashed across his broad, naked chest. Every dark shadow outlined his perfectly cut body in the most breathtaking way. Helplessly drawn to him like a moth to a brilliant flame, Ellora peered up at him through her thick lashes. She made no move to hide her brazen study as her eyes roved over him, examining the impressive build of the magnificent man who gazed down at her as if she were made of precious gold.

Little by little, Behr dragged his pants zipper down its track, letting them fall open in a painstakingly slow fashion, as if testing her level of comfortability, but succeeded only in heightening the tension that hung thick and heavy between them. Ellora's mouth ran dry as she watched him gradually pull them down his well-defined thighs before stepping out of them.

There he stood in all his glory, wearing nothing but the thin fabric of his formfitting boxer briefs, putting to shame any statue ever carved of the powerful Roman gladiators. Ellora's heart pounded inside her chest in anticipation. The fluttering of butterflies inside her stomach left her both anxious and nervous as he made his way back to her. The bed dipped under his impressive weight when he crawled over to her.

Behr hovered over his raven-haired girl, carefully gauging her reaction to his close proximity. Seeing his hesitation, Ellora pulled him impossibly close, desperately needing to quench the overwhelming need to have his arms wrapped around her.

He dragged his nose up the side of her neck, inhaling her intoxicating scent that had been driving his senses wild all night. His throat vibrated as he hummed in approval, the deep pulsating gyration causing Ellora's body to tremble with pent up desire. Behr ran his work-roughened hands up and down her quivering back, trying his best to sooth her.

"I'm right 'ere, love. Always right 'ere by your side. Nothing can keep me from you. I'm yours for the night."

Behr slid underneath the covers, smiling when she let out an adorable mewling noise as he sidled up next to her and wrapped his arm securely around her waist. He chuckled quietly as the adorable girl nuzzled into him, humming her appreciation. She fought against the pull of sleep as she lay peacefully in Behr's arms, while he placed kiss after kiss along the soft skin of her graceful neck. At his contact, she smiled ever so slightly, then curled up on her side. She drifted off to sleep in no time, her mouth slightly open in a small o.

Behr was lulled to sleep by the sound of her peaceful breathing. The best sound in the world.

Dalton waited until he was sure they were both completely

asleep. He quietly crept out of the shadows of his hiding place. He had been waiting there for the last few hours, watching, biding his time, to finally catch a moment alone with Ellora... waiting for the bastard to leave so the eager man could do to her what he had dreamed of since arriving in this town. To do exactly what that deplorable man was lucky enough to do right now.

His need to feel her soft body pressed against his, to savor her full lips, made his desperation escalate to unbelievable heights. He thought for sure after the movie, that the fucker would finally leave, but instead, he'd settled in for the night. Settled in her bed... right beside what belonged to him. His obsession was clouding the reasonable side of his brain, the thinking side. He had an overwhelming craving to slit his throat while he slept, but the thought of staining her porcelain skin with his repulsive, filthy blood stopped him from going through with the task.

Dalton would enact Behr's inevitable downfall soon enough. He would have to reconfigure his plans and come to Ellora on another night. The next time, he would definitely be alone with his emerald-eyed beauty. The smell of her delicate perfume beckoned to him, drawing Dalton closer to the vulnerable young girl.

He needed to test her lips before he left. It would hold him over for a while. He needed this. Just one caress from her delicious mouth and he'd leave. The snake crawled out from the protection of the shadows and inched his way closer to her sleeping form. He stealthily stalked across the old wood surface until he hovered over her bed.

His sinister smile grew as he stared down at her tempting body and curled, still form. That smile faded when his eyes adjusted on the ingrate's arm wrapped around the woman who belonged to him. It took all of his willpower not to rip the ape's arm off the object of his desire. Dalton kneeled down, settling a mere inches from her face.

His nose lightly skimmed down her cheek, neck, and collarbone. Ellora jumped a tiny bit at his touch. Inhaling the scent of her heated flesh, he shuddered as he blew the breath out. The whimper that escaped her lips almost pushed him over the edge. He wanted to hear her noises while he mounted and claimed everything her perfect body had to offer.

"Soon, my love. Very, very soon, I will feel the heat of your body wrapped tightly around mine." Ellora froze. Even her subconscious sensed when he was near. Dalton really liked that he had that lasting effect on her.

Slowly, he leaned in closer and brushed a feather-light kiss on her flawlessly enticing lips. "I'll be back for you. I promise." His tongue darted out to get a taste of her before he slithered back out the way he'd come in. The floor boards gave a haunting squeak, echoing in the quiet room as he left.

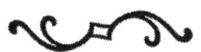

Ellora shot up, screaming. The vile sensation left behind from her frighteningly real nightmare still lingered on her trembling mouth. But that was impossible. Frantically looking around the eerily still room, her eyes glanced over her shoulder. Ellora did several double takes, shocked to see Behr reaching for her. To say she was relieved to see him was an understatement. That was some nightmare.

Ellora's breath was pumping in and out of her lungs rapidly, as she worked hard to regulate her erratic heart. "I swear, it was so real... I can still *feel* him here. I must be losing my mind."

"It's a'right, love. I'm 'ere. Nae another soul. You've just had a terrible nightmare. You're safe with me," he promised. Cupping her face in his hands, her protector stroked her tear stained cheek with his thumb. Ellora's eyes fluttered at his tender touch.

The frightened girl laid her head down on Behr's solid chest. Draping her hand over the impressive ridges of his sculpted abs, she blushed scarlet when she realized their limbs were still intimately entwined together. Gasping, she looked up into his eyes. "I fell asleep on you... didn't I?"

"Nae, love. You fell asleep, aye. But nae on me. Just think o' me as your own personal nightmare body guard."

The fear she experienced still lingered in the back of her mind, but faded away the longer she was in the presence of Behr's impossible to ignore pull on her heart. Ellora's shaking slowed down as she laughed weakly at his attempt to lighten the mood. "You can't defeat my nightmares, Behr."

He shook his head in disagreement. "Aaah, but I can, my love. I can chase those terrible dreams away for you."

Her fear faded away as she lifted a challenging brow in the dark. "Oh yeah? How can you do that? Inquiring minds want to know."

Hovering over her, Behr captured her bottom lip between his teeth just as her sentence ended, delighted to hear her gasp in surprise when he gave the plump flesh a good nip. The rumble of his laughter vibrated against her chest, awakening an urgent and deep seated need to have him closer, to have him possess her. All of her.

Ellora let her longing for him show as she pressed her eager lips to his, silently begging for the kiss she so desperately desired. Behr couldn't hold back any longer, delving into the heat of her waiting mouth and stroking her tongue with his in a rhythm that nearly drove her into madness. The dominant man deepened the kiss further, taking his time as he massaged the inside of her mouth, expertly sliding his tongue in and out. Behr gripped her delicate body. His strong hands pulled her hips closer. His desperation showcased his desire for her in an unmistakably intimate way as he ground his hips into her. His hypnotic undulations left her climbing higher and higher, losing herself in the ecstasy of the moment.

Knowing that she had been frightened and lay

completely vulnerable in his arms, Behr didn't want to take advantage of her by going too far. He gave just enough of himself to help her forget all her fears, which worked as he'd intended it to.

The sick and the eerie feeling that she was being watched faded into the back of her mind as Behr pulled her into pure bliss that she never wanted to come down from. Kissing away the leftover tears that wetted her cheeks, he whispered into her ear, "I've got you, love. I'm stayin' 'ere with you t' night."

Behr turned over in the bed and pulled his beloved with him, into his side. Ellora rested her head in the crook of his shoulder and wrapped her little arm over his waist. In no time at all, she drifted off to sleep.

The terrible nightmare she had woken up from was of past monsters taking Behr away from her. Permanently. This frightened her more than anything else, even more than her own safety. She didn't know what she would do without him, and the very thought brought a deep sadness into her heart. She tangled her legs with his and drifted off to sleep, comforted by his protective arms around her.

Ellora's last thoughts were of the man lying beside her, and before sleep claimed her once more, she whispered, "I love you, Behr. So much."

She needed Behr. She was complete as a person with him by her side, and after having lost so much already... She couldn't lose him.

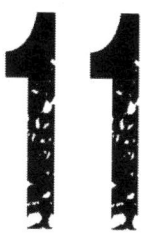

The long hours of night gave way to what promised to be an even longer day as dawn approached. Dominick and Giddeon sat on his homely worn old couch. The contents of the paperwork Susan surrendered to them was sprawled all over the coffee table. Only a handful of names remained on the list, dwindling their chances of finding a viable lead. They had worked through the night, looking at the list of names of all the unfortunate men who had worked for Dalton in the past.

After several calls, they ruled out job relocation, which Giddeon already knew wouldn't be a factor. They searched the internet for any possible residency change under their names or aliases, but were hit with many dead ends. Several of Dalton's former employees had been reported as missing by family members. Not a good sign.

Several more former secretaries had mysteriously vanished, as well. This case was growing out of the realm of anything Dominick had ever worked on before. Solving it would be tricky and would probably take more time than he had.

The detective was on the line with some guy he called

Tony, a man he trusted with his life, to run the remaining names. While he waited, Giddeon stared at his file. His gut churned and twisted with overwhelming sickness as the pale stranger glared back. Bile had him on the verge of expelling what little contents he carried, as he glared at the picture clipped inside. It was a picture of Giddeon a few years ago, and that person was unrecognizable.

The young man looked like a corpse; his zombie-like appearance shocked him. Pale skin and dark circles marred his otherwise youthful eyes, but the grief, anger, and bitterness had aged him. And those eyes... black, soulless, cold. The disheveled appearance that stared back at him was a disturbing wake-up call. Guilt and disgust with himself kept Giddeon from looking into mirrors for most of his life. What he envisioned in the mirror's reflection was enough to end his worthless life as past demons jumped out at him. He had to get this whole thing over with. Years of this had him slowly dying inside. He needed to either get busy livin' or get busy dyin', as they say. He was so ready to have this all be over, no matter the outcome.

Something in his file caught his attention, a notation clipped to some paperwork. Giddeon leaned in, unclipped the paper, and tried to read the scribbled pen note.

'In keeping a watchful eye on the boy, I'm delighted to see his darker nature progressing. I will set up a few instances to test out his instincts. Definitely keeping my eyes on this one. He could become quite useful to me in the near future. That is,

if he allows his inner demons to take over.'

What the fuck does that mean? Giddeon folded it back up and shoved it in his back pocket. The first time he'd ever seen Dalton was that day outside the club. Why was he talking about watching him as a boy? How did he know him? And where would he know him from?

Dominick ended the call, looking optimistic. Hopefully, someone had the man in the ballroom with the candlestick. Yeah, right. If life was a game of Clue, this shit would be a lot easier. Giddeon definitely thought there'd be a lot more action when the detective first told him he would help him take down Dalton. Not like *Forensic Files*, or *Law and Order* kind of action, but definitely a lot more action than he'd seen in the last few weeks. The most action he'd had was threatening Susan.

"Good news. This guy here was imprisoned just mere months after your parents' murders. He has been in and out ever since, on unrelated but just as violent crimes. He will be easily accessible since he can't get away from us. Let's head up there now and see what we can get out of him."

Giddeon shook his head in skepticism. "If this man is as hard as you think he is, he's not going to just tell you everything. He's already in prison. What more could we do to him that's not already been done? What would be his motivation or incentive to tell us what we want to know, Detective?"

"I've already thought about that. We'll take this file

and make him think that Dalton rolled over on him willingly when the law came sniffing around looking for Ellora. We'll tell him that Dalton and his high priced lawyers are spending a pretty penny gathering evidence on this man." Dominick waved the file in his hand, signaling the incarcerated man.

"We'll fib just a little and say the District Attorney is seeking a punitive penalty in the premeditative murders of Joseph and BonniBelle Sutherland, whose deaths we know were ordered by Dalton himself." Dominick smirked, confident in this plan. He folded his arms over his chest, waiting for more of his dark partner's cynicism, which followed immediately.

"I still think he will remain tight-lipped. What does he possibly have to lose?"

Dominick's smirk widened into a full-fledged, shit eating grin. "Ah, but he does. His latest four-year stint is over in a month's time. He can sense his freedom so bad, I bet he can almost taste it. Last thing he wants is life without the possibility of parole or the death penalty tacked onto his sentence. I think he will roll on Dalton, especially if we let him know that we are after Dalton from the start."

Giddeon unconsciously nodded, loving what he heard. "I like it, Detective. Nice work. Let's get out of here and talk to him then." Packing up the folder, Dominick grabbed his car keys and headed out for the drive down to the prison.

Security was pretty tight in the prison. They gave Dominick a hard time right out of the gate about wanting a room to interview Dale Nordin. Luckily, he was a persistent man and brought all the necessary documents and paperwork proving his status as a Detective. Giddeon wouldn't put it past Dalton to have a few inside men keeping an eye on his former employee. He just stayed quiet so that Dom could handle it, lest he ruin their chances. The guard announced that he was down the hall in a secured room, and to follow him.

Adrenaline flooded his system as he followed after him. Finally, he felt like they were getting somewhere. His heart pounded away inside his chest, hoping that they would get a chance to confront the man who might know where to find Dalton. Giddeon wanted to present the notation he found clipped to his file and see if this man knew anything about Dalton ordering a kid to be followed or watched all those years ago. He knew it was a long time ago and a longshot, but something didn't feel right.

Giddeon knew deep down that something was up, and he wanted to get to the bottom of it. Maybe since this man worked for Dalton around the same time, he'd have more of an insight into what his moves would be. Or, possibly, who the other men were who worked for Dalton, and where they had disappeared to.

That seemed like an awful lot of what-ifs.

The men were led down a gray concrete hallway, long,

narrow, and foreboding. Each step echoed louder and louder, giving the dark man a dreadful insight into the path he was on and soon to face. Shaking the feeling off just as soon as it had appeared, Giddeon put his game face on. He had a job to do.

Justice. Revenge. Peace.

After unlocking the door, the guard swung it open for them. Not too surprising, the con inside was older. His appearance was withered and disheveled from a long, hard life behind bars. His long, gray, scraggly hair was greasy and lay matted down. His life looked like it'd been a rough one, and his eyes revealed as much. Giddeon recognized his hardship at once. He understood.

The weary old man lifted his head up to see who was coming into the room, and Giddeon froze. The con was familiar somehow, but he couldn't seem to place him. Had Giddeon worked with him before?

Dominick cleared his throat and assumed a defensive stance. Giddeon laughed inwardly. *Cops.*

The con ignored Dominick completely. All of his attention lay focused on Giddeon, with the same confused recognition on his face. Without turning his head, Dale addressed the detective. "Thanks for getting me outta my cell, boss. So, I'm here. What can I do for you, Detective?"

Dominick sat in the comfortable desk chair he requested from the cell-block supervisor in charge, pulling the same shit he had on Giddeon when he was in Portree. Old habits die hard. Giddeon did his best to stand behind his mismatched partner, willing the guy into spilling his guts with the power of his imposing glare.

"Not sure if you've heard, but Dalton's crimes have all started to come back to bite him in the ass. One by one, his former employees have been rolling over on him, tired of his threats and black mail. We came here today hoping we'd get the same cooperation out of you." The man had a brief look of satisfaction wisp across his face. Then the confusion was firmly back in place.

"What do you want with me? I've been in here a long time. I haven't worked for Dalton for an even longer stretch of time."

Dominick leaned forward, ready to unleash his lie. "Ah, you see, Dalton has used his wealth to buy himself a fancy lawyer and a believable alibi."

The man nodded in disgust. "Of course he did, rat bastard."

The detective continued, happy that the man was playing right into his hands. "Well, he's stated to our D.A. that it had to be you. According to him, it went on behind the scenes without his knowledge, and you were the one behind all the illegal activities going on in his place of business. Namely, the attempted kidnapping and murder charges we want him for. He's making sure you take the fall for *his* crimes."

The convict cursed out, clenching his fists so tight the

knuckles turned a sickly white. "That's not possible. I've been in and out of here for a long time. I haven't been anywhere near that stupid prick in years. He's too twisted a freak to work with. I did one job for him and regretted it immediately, and every single day after that. Why me? What's his angle?"

Dominick tapped his folder on the table. "Well, you are the only one he could blame... Everyone else is missing. His high priced lawyer wants you for this, and they are working up quite a case on you. Turns out Dalton keeps very impressive, up-to-date files on anyone who's ever worked for him. He's very thorough."

The con pounded his fist on the table, his thunderous voice shouting his outrage as spit dribbled out of his sneering lips. "That's bullshit!"

"I know. Trust me, I know. We are here because we're the ones building the case *against* Dalton. I want to take him down. I know he's behind all of this. We just need your help."

Boy, Giddeon thought, Dominick sounded like a broken record. He'd spouted out this same shit at him in the Portree jailhouse.

"You see, all we have on him now are all these files, which do have his own personal notes on each of his former employees, including timelines and job descriptions. Unfortunately, that won't be enough to charge him with anything. It's all circumstantial. You, on the other hand, could wind up losing your whole life if you're wrongfully accused by a shark on the war path. You will be out of his way and stuck in this shithole for the rest of your life.

"That rat bastard will just continue obliterating the lives of others, untouched and as arrogant as ever. The more unstoppable he feels, the more dangerous he will become. Please, help us. Help yourself. You only have a month left. Don't let mistakes from your past dictate how you want to live your life in the future. You have the opportunity to right past wrongs... to dust yourself off and cash in on your second chance. Take it!"

Giddeon had to admit, the detective was really good at revving a person up and swaying him to see things in his perspective. Dominick looked back at him and asked, "Giddeon, can you get this man a coke or something? We're going to be here for a while."

The cuffed man whipped his head up at him, wide eyes protruding out of his paling face. The hardened criminal acted as though he'd seen a ghost. The bewildered scrutiny Dale directed at the marked man across the table from him was enough to unsettle even the hardest man's stomach. "No! It can't be. You're... You're not Giddeon... Giddeon Cane?"

Tremors shook his already on-edge body as warning bells went off inside Giddeon's throbbing head.

"How the fuck do you know who I am?" Giddeon stalked closer to the man, and Dominick wedged his body to stand in between them. "Just who are you? Why do you know me?" Giddeon asked again, malice laced thick in his rough tone.

Reaching into his back pocket, he snatched the now crumpled note Dalton had written and the old photo that was attached to Giddeon's file. Leaning as far as the table would allow, he raised them up inches from Dale's face. "Why was he following me?

The man looked like he'd walked right into a nightmare. His eyes were still wide and bulging out at Giddeon's towering presence before him.

"I... I was there. I was one of them. I didn't know it was going to happen like that until it was finished. We were supposed to just scare them out. That's what I'd been told. But, Dalton paired me with this psychopath."

The beast stirred inside of Giddeon. His eyes clouded over with a familiar red haze. Blinded by the rage that bubbled up inside of him, his frame shook with the effort it took to hold himself back.

Dominick pushed Giddeon down in his seat and stood over him, keeping a secure hand on his shoulder. "What are you talking about? Start from the beginning."

The convict was breathing like he'd just finished a marathon, almost gasping as he forced air into his lungs. It took him a minute to steady it enough to start talking.

"Dalton's first realty project was an artfully crafted building that was well over a century old and crumbling. He turned it into modern studio and two bedroom apartments.

It was a prime location. But, after all his work, he was told that he would only get the project off the ground if he provided off-street parking for the tenants."

Giddeon was getting extremely impatient with this story. It was taking too long. He just wanted the man to spit it out, to just tell him how he knew him. He was probably the man who Dalton had follow him.

"The only way he could do that was to relocate the people living in the rented townhouses that were unfortunate enough to sit directly beside the new building. Dalton was determined to go forward with the plan and wouldn't stop until he had his space.

"Dalton himself approached each family in private so there would be no record of his plan. He offered each tenant insane amounts of money to move, so long as they did so quickly. Dalton was getting impatient and frustrated because every family proclaimed that they would only move if one family in particular would move right along with them. They were well-liked and respected in the neighborhood."

Giddeon was confused as to how any of this had anything to do with him. "Get to the point, asshole!" he barked out at him. The sudden outburst made the man snap out of his story for a second. He looked directly at Giddeon with a sorrowful, gut-wrenching expression that someone wouldn't expect to see from a hardened criminal such as him.

"Your parents refused to sell, so the rest of their neighbors refused."

Giddeon was struck dumb. His gut already knew what was coming next, but he still found himself asking... hoping that the story would be different. "My parents?" His voice came out sounding small, insignificant.

The man forged ahead with the story, now in a rush to finish it. "Dalton figured that if one bad crime were to happen in the small community, the rest of the tenants would trip over themselves to take Dalton's money and leave. He knew the most respected group would be the ones who had to suffer his wrath. Once out of the way, there would be no more refusals. After all, Dalton always gets what he wants."

The marked man shook like an earthquake gearing up to unleash its devastating power on the unfortunate. His rage grew so overwhelming, Giddeon had no control over his body. It twitched and shook, every muscle coiling and tensing, ready to dispatch this man into the very hell he helped create. "It was you! It was YOU!" Giddeon shouted over and over.

Dale interrupted while Dominick held on to Giddeon, trying with all his might to keep him seated. "I had no intention of hurting anyone. The twisted man Dalton put me with couldn't wait to strike. I have thought of nothing else these past years but what happened to you and your parents. It has been a regret I have suffered with every single day since then." The man dipped his head in defeat.

Giddeon looked at him… studied him. He was the man who held on to his mother. His disgusting hands held her as the other man fought with his father. He remembered. This fucker wasn't off the hook, but Giddeon's need to get his hands on Dalton had just intensified even more. He'd ordered these men to kill his parents, but only one of them followed through with it… and it wasn't this man. He needed to find the other one.

Dominick, being the only man in the room who didn't know what happened next, asked, "What did you do to them?"

The man stayed quiet.

Giddeon's violently shaking body launched itself toward the cuffed convict across the table from him. Unable to keep Giddeon at bay this time, Dominick pushed against his advancing form. With tunnel vision, nothing and no one else existed to him, just the scraggily haired man in front of him. All the nightmarishly horrific scenes he'd witnessed as a frightened boy played back to him in slow motion. The look on his mother's helpless face as the dagger first made contact with her soft flesh was frozen in his consciousness.

Giddeon roared out, unable to contain his rage, easily throwing Dominick aside and catapulting himself over the table at the piece of shit who'd taken part in their murder. The force from the blow blew the cuffed man back, taking the heavy table with him. Once down, Giddeon rained punishing blows down on Dale's face, imagining it was all those years ago and wishing he'd been able to do to them then what he was able to do now. He wished he'd had the courage to fight the men, to stop them... to do *something*. As much as he willed his daydream to be enough to bring them back, he knew they never would. Nothing could bring them back.

Tears pricked the back of his unblinking eyes, and the sting brought him out of his wishful daydream to focus on the battered and bloody man underneath him. Dale didn't bother to fight him back. He hadn't even lifted a finger to shield his blows. The weathered and weary man just took it. Giddeon froze with his fisted hand in mid-air.

The man looked up at him, and with a strangled gurgling, spoke up with determination. "Do it. I deserve worse. I won't stop you."

Giddeon rocked back on his heels and sank to the floor, leaning up against the cold walls. His uttered statement knocked the wind out of him because *THAT* could be Giddeon. He had said this many times over. Staring at this emotionally broken man struggling to sit up with Dominick's help, he realized he was staring at his future. Dalton had turned this man's world upside down... destroyed Giddeon's life, and turned him into the very man he hunted down.

Dominick hollered over to his reckless partner, furious and confused about what had just transpired between the two. "Someone tell me what the fuck is going on… Giddeon? I'm about two fucking seconds away from locking you in here right along with him. How do you know him? What happened?"

All Giddeon's energy and will to fight back left his body, along with any feelings of rage he'd previously had. Utterly defeated, he bent over his knees and lay his head in his bloodied hands. With eyes pinched closed, he cast his mind back into a past that'd left him broken and numb. Mechanically, Giddeon relayed the story aloud.

"My mother and I were in the kitchen. She had been making me my favorite lunch of macaroni and cheese. My father had been in the front room watching fight prelims on the TV. Without warning, two men broke down the door, both wearing ski-masks, but they were not prepared to have my father jump up without hesitation and give them the toughest fight of their lives.

"They must not have done their homework because they weren't prepared to be fighting a boxer in his prime. Hearing the scuffle and shouts coming from the next room, my mother came running in and let out a terrified cry at the scene she witnessed. I followed but hid behind the end table. My mother continued to scream as my father warred with the masked men, gaining the attention of one of the fighting men.

"The bigger fighter shouted at the other, who seemed shocked that there was a woman and child at the house, to grab her. The piece of shit grabbed my mother and wrapped his arm

around her neck in a choke hold. She was my father's one and only weakness. Seeing the man with a knife to her throat took all the fight he had from him.

"The leader of the two men walked right up to my mother, and without a word or any lingering threats or hesitation, gutted her as she stood. Not satisfied with the carnage, he then slit her throat. This man let her drop to the floor where she bled out right in front of me. My father let a scream rip through him, a sound I'd never heard from him before. That sound still haunts me every night. He collapsed to the floor, lying next to the love of his life, staring in horror as her insides spilled out, and he just gave up.

"The man just kept stabbing my father as he lay with my dead mom, until he was satisfied that he was gone. They took off their masks and walked around trashing the place. When the monster found me hiding, he had a sick smile plastered on his blood spattered face.

"I froze. I thought for sure they would do the same to me. Violent tremors rocked through me. The man got down on one knee, pulled out his bloodied dagger, and placed the point of it under my chin. He forced me to lift my head with it so I could look evil in the eyes. He asked if I was going to avenge my parents, or do nothing and hide like a pussy.

He then grabbed my hand and confidently placed the dagger that was soaked with my parents' blood in my hands. He told me to do something about it. To avenge them. When I didn't move, he mocked me, saying, 'Yeah, that's what I *thought." His cruel, sinister laugh echoed through the apartment, and has echoed in my ears every day after that. Always right below the surface. Edging me closer and closer to madness."*

Dominick blew out an intense breath, while the convict sat running his hands through his hair, shaking his head. He swore he caught a glimpse of a few tears making their escape, but they were expertly hidden behind his curtain of scraggly hair.

"I didn't know he would do that. But that's no excuse. I should have stopped him. I know I should've stopped him." Dale chanted this a few more times, rocking back and forth.

Giddeon leapt at the man once more. "Shut the fuck up, you piece of shit!" He wanted to kill him, rip his flesh from his bones. He didn't expect that he would come face to face with one of the men responsible for ending their lives and ruining his. Several officers burst through the door to help assist Dominick in containing the outraged man.

Dominick repeated over and over, "He didn't do it. It was Dalton... Always Dalton. He ordered it, and the other man carried it out. We know now who it was. We just have to locate them... Giddeon, you finally know."

The cuffed man never even flinched, not even when Giddeon was a mere inches from striking his face. "Let him go, Detective. I deserve all the wrath this boy has toward me. I deserve worse. Let him go. I won't fight him."

Giddeon stopped short at his spoken words. Staring at

him, he realized that no matter how much he hated to admit it, Dominick was right. He wasn't the one who took his parents from him.

From twisted man to twisted man, Giddeon could tell that he was speaking the truth about not knowing. Dalton had used Dale, just like he'd used so many others to get what he wanted. The other piece of shit was the leader. He was the monster Giddeon remembered. And he would find him. He wouldn't stop until Dalton and that man were six feet under and rotting away. They were so close. It made him anxious to finally finish this. After all these years, Giddeon desperately needed to walk away from his torturous limbo he was stuck in and finally move on from it.

Dalton. How could he have done this? Why did he ask Giddeon to work side by side with him? He didn't understand why he would watch an utterly destroyed, emotionally messed up kid grow up, and then ask him to work for the very man who murdered his parents. But, he would ask him... in person, right before he watched him take his last breath. Looking over at his partner, he gritted out almost inaudibly, "Get me the fuck out of here NOW, before I lose my shit, Detective."

The cuffed man looked up, finally meeting the man's eyes whose boyhood face had haunted him his whole life. "I am truly sorry for every pain that we have caused you. I wish every single day that I could go back in time and change it, take it all back. I would in a heartbeat."

Giddeon pointed his finger at him. "Don't you dare think you're off the hook. I will be back for you."

The man nodded. "I know. And I'll be waiting."

Giddeon's anger grew even more. He didn't want him to be understanding. He didn't want him to accept his fate without a fight, because that wouldn't be the satisfying conclusion he'd always dreamed about. This was not at all how he thought this day would go, or how he'd expected a confrontation with one of the men would go. Giddeon was losing it bigtime. He had to get out of there quick; he needed to be alone where he could think. He desperately needed some perspective.

Giddeon told Dominick that he'd wait for him in the car. Dominick was relieved that he hadn't asked him to leave with him, because he still wanted some information from Dale. Dominick would use this terrible realization to wring information from him while he was still willing to cooperate. "Dale, what was the other man's name?"

The other man stared at the door Giddeon just left out of and responded, "Troy Wyndham. "

Dominick nodded. "Very good. Where can I find him?"

The man looked up at the detective. "I don't know. I've been in here. But I'd bet he is still working for him. Dalton just loves the twisted ones. He is extremely anal, and if you found my file in his possession, I'd bet his is in there somewhere. That's the best I can tell you. You have a name. All you need is the information. I could tell you where he liked to hang out, or places he liked to eat, but like I said before, I only pulled one job with him. I never wanted any of this. I'm just a thief, not a murderer. I'm not a murderer."

Dominick watched him as he started chanting and rocking again. This was something that had obviously affected him because, since the moment he laid eyes on Giddeon, his demeanor had regressed immediately.

"All right, thank you for your cooperation. I'll be back when I have him for your positive identification. I think it's about time we give Giddeon back his life. Don't you?" The withered man dropped his head in his hands, drowning in the memories of an unforgiveable past.

Dominick walked out of the holding cell. This had really knocked him on his ass. This was not at all what he was expecting would happen when they arrived. But, at least they had two names. One they knew, the other they hadn't. Now, they just had to locate them both. Yeah, that was easier said than done. But, at least they were a few steps closer than when they started out that morning.

Developing a new sense of urgency in trying to locate Dalton, Dominick realized he was far more dangerous and ruthless than he had originally thought. He would go to Susan and offer her protection if she helped them out and disclosed where he was hiding. That is, if she even knew. He hoped to God that she did. The longer he was on the run, free, the more risk there was of someone else falling victim to the unstoppably evil man.

Taking his time walking to his car, the detective had half expected Giddeon's ankle monitor to go off, but it never did. He sat in the passenger seat, staring ahead at nothing in particular. Once Dominick was in the car, Giddeon announced much too loudly for the tight space, "I need to go somewhere. It's um, it's really important. Please. Don't ask me any questions, okay."

Dominick was silent for a few minutes, then finally answered, "Where to?"

"215 North State Street."

Once Dominick punched the address into his GPS and recognized where that was, he lifted an eyebrow. This man kept surprising him, in a good way. He hated that this kid kept growing on him. He was cut a raw deal in life. But, he didn't want to forget his crimes altogether, just because he had compassion for him. He had to keep reminding himself that.

"All right, Giddeon, how long do you want to be there? I'll punch it into the ankle monitor's list of acceptable locations besides group." Having no more will to speak, Giddeon just nodded, leaving the question unanswered.

It finally dawned on Dominick what day it was and the reason behind Giddeon's odd request. "I'll give you the day, all right? If you're ready to go sooner, just call my cell."

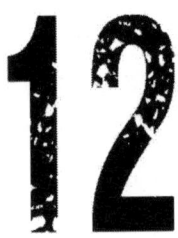

Giddeon walked through the massive cathedral doors of Saint John the Evangelist Catholic Church. Gripping his mother's rosary, he marched halfway up the aisle and sat in a lovingly used pew. The church was thankfully quiet, its vacant state mirroring the emptiness that dwelled deep inside his aching chest. Bowing his head, Giddeon recited a few prayers from memory, begging for guidance, mercy, and forgiveness. He reflected on all the events leading up to his parents' murders, the recent events that brought him there on his knees, and everything in between. His arms leaned on the pew in front of him, successfully hiding his face and the tears that trickled down into his five-o-clock shadow.

Today had been a devastating shock to his system. Old wounds ripped open in his chest, leaving him vulnerable and exposed for the world to see. Even after all this time had passed, the anguish was too much to bear. The boy who'd been left behind to suffer through all the traumatic aftermath, all alone, had been morphed into the very monster he was after. He never meant to turn into this heartless, uncaring *thing*.

He longed to wrap his arms around his mother and see the proud look that his father used to give when he taught him something new. Too much time had passed. His parents wouldn't even recognize their own son, even if they were standing right there in front of him. He could almost sense their disgust at the vile, unfeeling animal he'd turned out to be.

The emotionally disturbed man was so tired of being stuck in limbo; Hell would be a vacation compared to the torment he'd suffered here on earth. Giddeon was tired of going it alone. He was tired of fighting. It was all just compensation for the one battle he should have fought. The only one that mattered all those years ago.

Giddeon sat on the hard wooden bench, surrounded by a sea of old tattered padding in the familiar cathedral. He'd always remembered it as full of people, full of life, and full of joy. Now, just like him, it resembled a dark, solemn, and hollowed out shell. He longed to feel the presence of their spirits in his heart, or sense their presence surrounding him. But he didn't. He felt nothing. That was the worst of it all. Numbness. Nothingness.

Giddeon squeezed the rosary tighter as he whispered brokenly, "I'm so sorry I didn't fight for you, Mama... I'm so sorry I didn't protect her, Dad. Please, forgive me." His chest caved in on itself like a heavy weight was crushing down on him. It was excruciating to breathe.

"The path I've been on has led me so far from you

both, so far from what you taught me. Past demons have stolen my sanity. I've held on to anger and revenge for so long, I don't know how else to be. Please. If you haven't already turned your backs on me, help lead me onto the correct path. I don't even know where that is anymore." Giddeon marked the sign of the cross—head, chest, and shoulder to shoulder—before standing.

Forcing himself up on weak, unwilling legs, he made his way up to light a few candles in the front of the sanctuary. Lifting his weary head, he noticed a familiar blonde sitting a few pews up. He hadn't noticed her when he first walked in. He sauntered up to where she sat and sidled in right next to her. She was deep in prayer. Her eyes were pinched shut. Something was worrying her.

He was tempted to reach out and smooth out the stress lines on her forehead with his thumb. She hadn't even realized that someone had sat down directly next to her. It could've been the Devil himself, and she didn't seem to care. Without even opening her eyes, she spoke up, "Hello, Giddeon. What are you doing here?"

The broken man cracked a smile which seemed to always be reserved for her. "How'd you know it was me, Angel?"

It was her turn to smile. The worry lines melted away, leaving behind flawless porcelain skin. When her eyes opened, they reunited with Giddeon's. She was taken aback by his appearance. He seemed to have aged ten years since his short time away from her. Her dark knight was withered, pale, and wore black circles under each eye. Even though he smiled, Eva could see the haunted look in his eyes. She wasn't fooled; something significant had happened. She knew this look well. She had worn it so many times before, when she was moments away from giving up.

Eva finally answered Giddeon's question after they both took time looking each other over. They both appeared a little worse for wear. "I could smell you before you even came near me. Your shampoo and soap together give you a certain smell that my senses picked up on." That was kind of the truth, but really, her body sensed everything about him and automatically knew when he was close by. She was helplessly drawn to him and wasn't really surprised that they'd ended up in the same place.

Even though Giddeon missed group that day, Eva prayed she'd still see him. The need to know he was doing okay grew as time ticked by at an agonizingly slow pace. Try as she might, she couldn't *NOT* think about him. He was always in her thoughts, and she couldn't help but be concerned for him when he was out of her sight. From the moment she woke until the time her head hit the pillow at night, this dark and broken man had claimed all her thoughts. He was holding on to such a gruesome, devastating past, and Eva was compelled to protect him from any further tragedies.

Giddeon stretched his arm out behind her on the back

of the pew. "What are you doing here, Angel? Everything all right?" He ignored her very same question and threw it right back at her. He had to know that she was okay. She looked worried, like the weight of the world rested on her delicate shoulders. He knew very well what that was like, and he didn't want her feeling that way. His Angel deserved nothing but happiness.

"Oh, well, I still have my tough days that I have to fight through just to make it to the end. On those days, I come here. This place always puts me at peace. My grandmother used to bring me here for mass. I guess this is what gave my mom and dad the idea for my name."

Giddeon leaned back and studied her face. He wanted to make sure she wasn't making it up for his benefit. No. There's no way she'd do that. She was brutally honest. Plus, Dominick didn't even know that this was the church his mother attended until he'd given him the address that very morning. "My mother used to bring me to mass here, too. Every Wednesday and Sunday, without fail." Giddeon grasped the beloved rosary and kissed it unconsciously. Glancing down with nothing but devotion for the precious reminder, he rubbed it lovingly between his rough, calloused hands. Every time he closed his eyes, he could still visualize his beautiful mother clutching the very same beads in her delicate hands.

The action caught Eva's attention. "Is that hers? It's beautiful." Reaching out, she lightly fondled the artfully crafted beads that hung low on his chest.

Giddeon gasped, unsure of how to take her sudden response. He wouldn't have dared let anyone else in the world touch them. Before he could figure out how he felt about that, she let them go and gazed up at him. Her beautiful blue eyes stole away his breath.

"What are you doing in here, Giddeon? You look like you're having a day that rivals mine. What's up?" Her voice was a soft whisper, but the grand empty cathedral still managed to bounce her words around the immense archways in the massive sanctuary. For a moment, he hesitated. He had always hated talking outside of the confessional, like all of the statues were staring at him... Judging him. Their eyes always seemed to find you anywhere in the room.

Taking a deep breath in, he ran his hands through his floppy hair. Her eyes darted all over his face attentively, ready to listen. Her concern touched him in a dark forgotten place in his heart. "I... I always come here. Every year. On the same day."

Giddeon had hoped that she'd pick up on the not so subtle hint, but her confusion was written in her raised brow and curious expression, so he pressed on. "This is the anniversary of their murders. I always feel close to my mother when I'm here. This time is different, though. Today is different."

Giddeon stopped the story right there. He just didn't

know how to reiterate everything he'd found out that morning. His mouth opened and shut several times before he gave up and faced forward. She wouldn't want to know. His life was utterly depressing and pathetic. Why did she keep looking at him like he was worth something more? She shouldn't be hanging out with a dangerous *monster* like him. He'd just drag her down into his despair.

Eva bit her lip in concentration. She waited for an unknown amount of time for him to finish, but he never did. His brokenness tugged at her heart, causing it to ache with a deep sadness for him. "What is so different about this time, Giddeon? We are all alone in here. You can trust me."

The reluctant man shook his head defiantly. "No. You don't want to know any more about my fucked up life. It's better if you don't. You shouldn't even be sitting here with me. You should stay away from me."

Eva grabbed hold of his chin and forced him to look at her. "I don't want to hear you talk like that again. Not to me. I have suffered with my own demons. I still do. I am no better and no worse than you or anyone else." She leaned in so close, her lips were just a breath away. It caused his nerves to wake up and jump in awareness. She always had this effect on him. His Angel always managed to rouse his dead body with an exhilarating jolt.

"And neither are you," she added. "Now, tell me, or I will find a way to dig it out of you. I'm stubborn enough to do it, too." She lifted a challenging brow. Giddeon definitely believed that statement. "And, besides, I was here first. You came over here and sat down in my pew, remember?" Her lips twitched as they smirked in the most tantalizing way. What a cute little smart ass. He was tempted to bite the arrogant lip that teased him.

"I guess in that, you're right. But it is still your fault." Giddeon looped his finger around a glimmering golden lock, wrapping it around his fingertips.

Eva looked incredulous at his accusation. "How do you figure that?"

Giddeon was both shocked and captivated that, unlike every other time he'd played with her hair, she didn't pull back or yank it away. She let him continue to run his fingers through the waves. Her hair was so soft and silky. He could run his hands through it all day. "It's not my fault you draw me to you like a beacon. I'm helpless against your pull."

He was shocked by the words that just spilled out of his mouth, as if by their own will, while absentmindedly playing with the loose strands. And by the look on his precious Angel's face, so was she. The same hand that was running through her hair reached up and cupped her blushing cheek, his thumb lightly stroking the pink skin.

She closed her eyes and sighed. "Oh, Giddeon. What are you doing to me?"

"I'm not doing anything you aren't already doing to me, Angel," Giddeon whispered back.

"That may be true, but I'm not so easily swayed. What

has changed? Why is today so different, Giddeon?" The stubborn girl smirked when the man she was helplessly drawn to tugged on the lock of hair he held captive.

The melancholy figure that sat so close beside her sighed heavily. He turned forward in the pew, away from the prying eyes that captivated him. Eva was disappointed when their shared connection had switched off, following his shift in position.

Giddeon was once again cold and expressionless. She wanted nothing more than to wrap her arms around him and show him what love could feel like. That was so incredibly messed up, because she was supposed to be helping him, but she couldn't stop imaging what it would be like to wrap herself around him. To feel his weight as it came down on hers.

Against all her warnings and self-promises, Eva was in serious danger of falling for Giddeon Cane. She shook her head of those dangerous thoughts. They were definitely *not* helping right then.

"Dominick and I went to the prison to interview one of Dalton's ex-employees to see if he had any idea where he might be hiding himself." There was an incredibly long pause. Something significant must've happened, because Giddeon was struggling with himself, trying hard to keep his composure. He clenched his hands together in tight fists and rested them on the pew in front of him.

Eva's heart broke for him when he dipped his head

182

low. He was breaking. This wasn't good. Eva went against the screaming in her head that urged her to listen and keep her distance. Instead, she went with her breaking heart and wrapped her arms around him, placing tender kisses along his throbbing temple. He stiffened under her delicate embrace. She somehow brought him out of his thoughts and back to his current reality.

"He... he was one of the men there that day. He was there, Eva. After all these years I've waited to come face to face with one of these bastards, and I just walked away. I have planned for years what I'd do if I ever got a chance to get my hands on one of them." Eva was taken aback when he turned his glare on her. His eyes had dilated all the way, appearing unnaturally black, giving him a frighteningly demonic expression. The void of color, warmth, and light raised goosebumps on her trembling arms.

He turned, facing her, and stared unblinking down at her. "I should've killed him right there. I should've punched my blade into his gutless flesh and spilled his blood all over the dirty floor, just as they had done to my parents, but... I... I just couldn't. I froze. Just like all those years ago, I froze and did nothing. I'm a worthless coward. They should've ripped me wide open and exposed me for the weakling that I am, and just let me die along with them. I deserve it. They didn't."

The stranger sitting next to her finally tore his gaze away from her and ducked his head. This was the raw emotion she was trying to get out of him in group, and now that she'd seen it, she immediately wanted to amend it. She wasn't surprised that he blamed himself. But, her heart ached to hear him say it, longing to comfort him.

"Giddeon. You were only six years old. What could you do? You survived. That's what your parents would have wanted, and that's what kind and loving parents are supposed to do... protect their children." Giddeon snapped his head up at her. His murderous glare startled her for a brief second as it cut right through her mid-sentence. She stopped talking.

"They would never have wanted me to survive if they laid eyes on me now, saw who I truly am. If they'd witnessed the things I've done..." He reached into his pocket and pulled out a large dagger.

"I. Am. A. Monster."

For some absurd reason, Eva wasn't scared. She should have been, but she wasn't. Looking down at the deadly object in his palm, she couldn't help but ask, "What's that for, Giddeon?"

The now unrecognizable man sitting next to her glowered at the deadly weapon in his hands. "This is the dagger they used to gut my parents."

Eva regarded the terrifyingly intimidating piece, then reluctantly asked, "Why... why do you have this, Giddeon? Why would you carry that around with you?"

Turning it over several times, he ran his fingers along

the faded emblem on the handle. "I just stood there. As my parents' souls were savagely ripped out long before their time, I... I just stood there and did nothing." Giddeon fondled the sharp edge of the blade, pressing it into the roughened pad of his fingertip.

"One of the men stalked over to where I lay hidden, and presented this dagger to me. It was covered in their blood. He challenged me to avenge them. He actually grabbed my hand and placed it in my palm. Even with the weapon, I still did nothing. Like a coward, I just laid there, frozen on the spot.

"I've kept this dagger with me every single day since then, to remind me that my hesitation and fear is what killed my parents. Not those men. I should've fought them... I should've done *something*. Instead, I just sat there and watched."

Eva's eyes were tearing up. This man had suffered so much. "Giddeon, no matter what you've built up in your mind... You. Where. Only. Six. Giddeon, you were a child, and you suffered far worse than they did. You had to watch. You've had to carry this unbelievable burden around with you as you grew. No one has been in your corner to support you. You've been living in a real life nightmare that you can't seem to dig yourself out of. None of this has been your fault. You were just a child. It is very obvious that you are suffering from PTSD."

"Isn't that like what men in the armed forces get after

war?" Giddeon forced out, incredulous.

Eva nodded. "You are a danger to others and most importantly yourself. Because of your neglected childhood, you were never diagnosed. You've never had someone in your corner looking out for you. It's never too late to seek help. It's never too late to start living your life, Giddeon. I am here for you. I will help you in any way that I can."

"What makes you think I have that?" The denial was on his face and clear in his tone.

"Oh, I know you have that." Eva shot him a 'just try and argue with me' look. "Anyone can suffer from PTSD. It's a mental health condition triggered by seeing or experiencing a terrifying event. You show all the signs—you experience terrible nightmares, flashbacks, aggression, and self-destructive behavior. And you'd have to be Superman if you didn't after everything you've suffered through."

Giddeon shook his head in disbelief. "Then cure me. You've solved the mystery, Velma. Where's my magical blue pill that will turn my fucked up world into shining rainbows? Hook me up."

Eva blew out a frustrated breath and mentally prepared herself for a battle of wills. Most of the group members she'd come into contact with acted like this when someone said they could help. Life's cruel events were the root of their extreme skepticism.

"This is a condition that can't be cured, but treatment can help you. Keep going to group therapy sessions, and have a doctor properly diagnose you so he can prescribe the proper medication to help you. It will get better with time. I will stand by you, through it all, Giddeon. Whether you want me to or not." Eva lifted a challenging brow and smirked at the hard-headed man.

"What if I don't want to be cured? What if I feel the most in control when I'm...? What did you call it again? Oh, yeah, self-destructive and violent. What if I'm just twisted? Simple as that. Better get used to that, Angel. Some people can't be patched up good as new by a doctor's note and talking to a group of strangers."

Eva once again captured his full attention by climbing up onto his lap, straddling him. "Oh, Giddeon, that's where you are so wrong." She grabbed his face roughly with both hands and forcefully lifted his head, so he had nowhere else to look but in her eyes. She would get through to him. She didn't care how she had to do it, or how unorthodox the method. He deserved to finally start living his life. He deserved peace.

"You don't have control. You never did. That's an illusion you've let yourself believe after all this time. Those monsters have you trapped in the prison they've created for you. They are the ones who've had control all along, ever since that day. They have controlled you all your life."

Giddeon's face hardened in her hands, growing rigid with anger. "No. No one controls me..."

Eva shocked her dark warrior by softly kissing his

mouth, successfully shutting him up. " Giving up on life... allowing the grief and unbearable guilt you feel take over you like this, is *exactly* what those monsters wanted. The moment you gave in to your despair and let it wreck your own life, they won. They have ultimate control over you when you let that happen. Don't you see that? I know it feels better in the heat of the moment to give in to your anger, to give in to the beast that seduces you into releasing the pain temporarily... But it is catastrophic to the spirit. It imprisons you.

"Getting past that guilt and grief is the hardest thing you'll ever have to do. But, once done, the incredible feeling you get from it is freeing. Only then will you have ultimate control over your life. I know it seems impossible now, but once you hit rock bottom, you can only go up from there."

Once again, she softly placed a feather-light kiss on his frozen lips, then got up abruptly. Reaching out her hands to her wounded warrior, she silently beckoned him to follow her.

Still in shock from the unexpected kiss, Giddeon's body stood on its own accord and sidled up next to his very own guardian angel. "Where are we going?"

Eva tugged on his hand and marched down the aisle and out the doors. "We are going to my place. I'm making you dinner. How long has it been since you've had a home cooked meal?"

Giddeon struggled with that question. He thought

hard, wanting to prove her wrong by coming up with an answer, but couldn't.

"That's what I thought. C'mon. My place is right across the street."

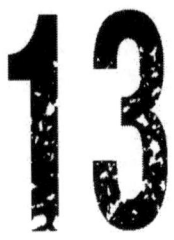

After Dominick dropped off Giddeon, he made a bee-line for Susan's place of residence. He had looked it up, hoping to catch her before she went into work, knowing that her every move was probably being watched while they were there. She would most likely feel safer talking to him in the comfort of her own home. He knew she was aware of Dalton's whereabouts, and he needed to dig it out of her. Dominick grew more and more anxious to find him. How many more lives had he destroyed? His malicious intent seemed unending.

Exhausted, he pulled up to her tiny townhome. The heavy SUV crunched the loose gravel of the unpaved driveway as he came to a stop. Blowing out a weary breath, the detective pulled the keys out of the ignition. It was now or never. Skipping up the stone steps and jingling his keys anxiously, the on-edge detective rang the bell. He said a silent prayer that the scared woman wouldn't slam the door in his face, and that she'd tell him what he wanted to know.

Light footsteps padded closer to the door, and after a long pause, heavy deadbolts were pushed aside and a chain-lock removed. The door opened a hairline crack, and a pair of scared, beautiful eyes peered out at him. It took Dominick a minute to realize that the woman standing before him was, in fact, Susan.

She looked like a completely different person. Her hair, no longer in a smooth, tight, up do, hung in loose waves down her back. The laid back style looked like she had just come back from a carefree day at the beach. She had on a fitted t-shirt and purposely torn and faded jeans. This down to earth persona called out to him in an unsettling way.

To say that Dominick appreciated this look on her was an understatement.

"Detective Antonelli? How can I help you?" She nervously inspected up and down both sides of the street. Her stance shifted from one foot to the other, obviously worried about being caught talking to the detective.

"I have some more questions I want to ask, and I figured it was safer for you if I came here, instead of showing up at Dalton's high-rise... again. May I come in?"

The distrustful girl asked, "You... you didn't bring Giddeon here... did you?"

Dominick shook his head. "No. I would never do that."

She hesitated for a brief moment, biting her lip, then stepped aside. She opened the door wide enough to let him pass, and then quickly closed it behind him, locking the dead bolts back up as if by trained habit. This woman lived her life in constant fear. Dominick realized that she must've witnessed horrifying occurrences while working as Dalton's secretary.

"Could I get you something to drink? Some coffee?" Susan motioned for the detective to follow her lead.

Dominick nodded and followed the beautiful but edgy girl as she padded barefoot into her elegant kitchen. Unable to help himself, he appreciated the way her tight jeans hugged every curve affectionately, and the glimpse of soft flesh revealed through the scattered tatters that worked their way up each thigh.

"That'd be great, Susan. Thank you." She motioned for him to sit at the quaint little kitchenette table as she went about preparing his coffee.

He watched with fascination as she pulled out all the stops, even going as far as boiling the milk into a rich frothy cream. Dominick had a Keurig, which made for weak, watered down coffee, and the coffee at the station was sludge. He was used to it, but the aroma Susan's coffee gave off had him salivating as it hung rich and thick in the air.

He couldn't help but ask as he watched in fascination as she strained the milk into the dark brew and slid the thick frothy cup his way, "Do you always take this much time and care into making one cup of coffee?"

Susan smiled ever so slightly as she sat down in the ladder back chair across from him. Dominick marveled at her brilliant white teeth, realizing that this woman didn't seem to smile all that often. It gave him one more reason to despise Dalton even more. This woman needed to be free of him. "My grandmother swears by this method. It tastes so much better than artificial creamers, and it's worth every effort. This process of making coffee was handed down to my mother, then to me."

Dominick took care inhaling the rich decadent aroma. "Mmm, this smells delicious. Thank you, Susan." Lifting an eyebrow in waiting, Susan watched as he took a sip, taking care not to burn himself, waiting for his assessment. "Oh my God, woman! You've got to be kidding me." The authoritative man moaned, rolling his eyes back into his head. "What kind of coffee is this?" he questioned in awed reverence at all the mouthwatering flavors swirling around in his mouth.

Once again, the stunning woman smiled at him, this time a little wider as she enjoyed watching him take pleasure in her coffee. "It's called Café Bustelo. It's a dark espresso roast, my personal favorite."

Dominick unceremoniously sucked it down in greedy gulps, not caring in the least that it scalded the roof of his mouth. "I think I'm in love." He couldn't help but gush.

Susan laughed light and heartily at his appreciative display. The melody reminded him of the subtle wind chimes his grandmother had that sang with the breeze on a hot summer day. It was music to his ears.

"I get that all the time. Once, I even received a marriage proposal. It's the reason Dalton first hired me. I was working as a waitress at the diner in Franklin Square, and was quickly put in charge of the coffee at his office after he had sampled one of mine." She shrugged, her smile disappearing. The eyes that had been full of life and laughter just seconds before suddenly glossed over as she was cast into a dark daydream.

Dominick took in the sight of her and nodded his head in understanding. "He is the reason I've come here to see you today."

Susan closed her eyes and whispered wearily, "I figured as much."

Dominick knew he was risking her safety by being there, and he knew she thought the same way. "Dalton is going down, one way or another."

Susan nodded, pinching the bridge of her nose, and managed to ground out, "I knew it was a matter of time... I just wish it hadn't taken this long to catch up to him."

"I'm truly sorry. If I'd known, I would've come to get you out sooner. Dalton is very good at keeping his employees silent by imprisoning you with fear. But, I'm here now. Because of Joseph, his head foreman, we are building quite a case against him. He sent detailed documents of his extensive criminal activity over to his lawyer before he was murdered. The documents date back to include a decade's worth of illegal activities ordered under Dalton's authority.

"We have Ellora's testimony, along with his hired gun, Dale Nordin, and Giddeon Cane, all of whom are ready and willing to take him down. I don't want you getting caught up in the crossfire. I don't want you getting dragged down with him. That seems to be his style—letting others catch the fall. It is all about winning to him. Even if he's caught, he will try to ruin as many lives as he can."

Susan began worrying her lip at the heavy weight of his words. Unable to stop himself, Dominick reached out and released her lip from the punishment of her teeth with the pad of his thumb. He grasped hold of her trembling hands and went on.

"I came here for two reasons. First, because I know you alone know of Dalton's whereabouts. And second, to offer you protection for your testimony."

Susan quaked at the mention of going up against the ruthless, unstoppable evil that held all that she loved in this world captive. She risked a frightened glance at the detective across from her. The terrified expression that passed over her pale face reminded him of what had happened to Vicky. Helping him would put her life at risk. And he couldn't let that happen... again.

More determined than ever to keep this girl safe, he vowed to keep a close personal eye on her. Dominick had to restrain himself from bringing the terrified girl into the comfort of his protective arms.

"Do... do you mean witness protection?" Her tiny voice quivered as she tried her best to look stronger than she was.

He nodded. "Yes. I want to keep you safe. I *WILL* keep

you safe, Susan. He will no longer control you. You will have no reason to fear him any longer."

She shook her head adamantly. Her eyebrows dipped, showing her serious concern. "I've never been frightened for myself. I don't care what happens to me." Hesitating for a moment when Dominick glared at her, Susan weakly demanded, "Promise me that they'll be safe. I want it in writing. Swear to me that Dalton won't be able to touch them, and I'll tell you anything you want to know." Susan began chewing on her abused lip once more. "Protective custody is when you're given a new identity, new job, and new life... right? No one will know of our whereabouts, right?"

Dominick nodded sternly. "Yes, only a select few will know who you really are, and where you are. I will see this through, Susan. You have my word. I'll keep you safe."

The determined girl waved her hand dismissively at his statement, once again assuring him, "I'm not worried about me. I told you, I'm worried about my mother and little brother. Dalton has, on more than one occasion, threatened me with *their* lives. I don't work for him because I want to... I work for him because I *HAVE* to. Dalton's left me with no other choice. Their health and well-being rest solely in his hands."

Dominick brought his hands up, trying to pacify the now hysterical girl panicking before him. He watched as tears spilled over the corners of her eyes.

"It's okay. Tell me what's going on. I want to help get you out. You can trust me." Tears continued to roll down her cheeks as she willed herself to trust this brave man who was willing to take on the Devil himself.

"My mother is in a top notch hospital with gold star treatment. She suffers from an advanced case of dementia. Her symptoms started early on in life, and then a few years ago, she got to where I could no longer care for her all by myself. She was a handful. Dalton swooped in and sunk his claws into me, offering to put her up and fund her stay, so long as I worked for him.

"His offer seemed so generous at the time. Once he found out that my little brother, Alex, is a special needs child, he shipped him away to the best school available, where he's receiving round the clock care. It's all paid in full, courtesy of Dalton Ramsey Claiborne himself. He became the master of my life and has owned me every single day thereafter. If I go… they have to come with me."

Yanking her hands from his tender touch, she crossed them over her chest. She stared at Dominick with a stubborn willfulness, daring him to deny her demand. Dumbfounded by the unexpected story, he wondered how many more lives Dalton had under his thumb. How many lives had he ruined? Shaking his head of that horrifying thought, he addressed the selfless girl sitting before him.

"They are immediate family, so I'm sure the District Attorney will have no problem with that. I will have them both signed over to you as their primary care giver. I'll make a call to their office now and have the paperwork rushed. Do you have a fax machine? I think we can push to have this hashed out by tonight." Susan nodded, ready for the change, and thankful for the opportunity to break free from Dalton's tight grip on her life.

Life. What a joke. This had been a prison sentence, and her time was now up. Thank God. "Yes, Detective. I'm in. Set it up now, and I'll tell you everything."

Twelve hours later, late into the evening, all the deals where approved, and all the details had been hashed out. The D.A. interviewed Susan via live web cam to save everyone some time. Now, she was tirelessly signing a mountain of paperwork. No going back now. The deal had already been set into motion. "What happens to my mother and brother now?"

Dominick scooped up all the papers, dialed the appropriate numbers into the fax machine, and began feeding all the documents to the D.A.'s office. "We already have an agent en-route to pick them up and take them to your new location. You can join them as soon as we are through here. They each will have a trained and licensed nurse to help you with their care. You're free now, Susan. You can finally breathe easy."

Closing her eyes, she allowed herself to breathe deeply for the first time in a very long time. Lifting her head, she sighed. "Thank you, Dominick. Thank you from the very bottom of my heart." With one more deep cleansing breath, Susan stood up and walked with purpose over to a filing cabinet hidden inside the corner of her tiny office closet. Thumbing through several file folders, she stopped at one and pulled it out.

With renewed strength, the determined girl walked over to join the detective. For the first time that day, she was able to look him right in the eyes. Sucking in a deep breath, Susan steadied her nerves while blowing the rest out forcefully… finally ready to tell all.

Knowing that this was extremely difficult for the girl, Dominick did his best to ease her fears. "It's okay. Take your time, sweetheart." Dominick didn't mean to let the endearment slip from his lips, but once uttered, he had to admit to himself that he was attracted to the girl. The thought of her leaving and never coming back left him feeling hollow inside.

Every time he let himself even think he might be able to start something with a woman, she was soon after ripped away from him. Dominick appreciated the beauty of her eyes for a little while longer while Susan collected her thoughts. They were a rich hazel with almost transparent green flecks in them. When she finally cleared her throat, he quickly glanced away.

"These are all the files of Dalton's ex-employees that he wanted dispatched when they displeased him in one way or another. He hired men to make sure that happened. I'm not sure where or what was done to them, but I'm sure you all can investigate that." She handed them over slowly.

Dominick gripped them, then slowly pulled them out of her trembling hands. "Why'd you hang on to these, Susan?"

Lifting her head in defiance, she declared in a stern voice, "Dalton's not the only one who can blackmail. I was collecting them, hoping I could find someone to pass them off to... someone I could trust. A man who wasn't under Dalton's control. I've dreamed of breaking free from him for a very long time, Detective, just biding my time, serving my sentence under his rule. Waiting for the day I'd be freed."

Shaking his head at the desperately distraught girl, he couldn't imagine what her life must've been like working for that bastard. "That was very brave, risky, and incredibly stupid of you, but I'm glad you did it. For both of our benefits." They both let out a forced laugh.

Susan allowed herself one good appraisal of the detective who'd come to her rescue. He was handsome, domineering, and a very brave man. His physique was in fine shape, most likely a requirement for the job he took so seriously. She appreciated his impressive masculine features and smirked at him, wishing that she'd met him under different circumstances.

"Well, someone had to do something, no matter how small, to try to stop him before he ruined more lives." Her blonde waves bounced as she shook her head in disgust. "I just wish I could've done something sooner. I was horrified by what happened to Ellora's father, Joseph. He was a really kind and wonderful man, always very respectful."

She stopped mid-sentence, parting her perfectly glossed lips, and hesitated for a second before continuing. "And that brings me to this file." Susan placed the folder in the detective's waiting hands.

Glancing down, his eyes bulged at the words as they stared back at him. "What's all this? Where is he?"

She bounced her knee up and down nervously. "The day you caught Giddeon, Dalton booked a flight out to Scotland the next day. He acquired a car and property there. He has been there ever since. He hasn't come back, not that I know of anyway."

Dominick pulled out his phone immediately. "That was months ago! He's got his sights set on Ellora. He won't come back without her. Fuck! She's in serious danger."

Susan's trembling intensified, and she began to bite her fingernails roughly, not knowing what else to do. "I'm sorry. I didn't know who to tell. I didn't know who I could trust."

Pacing the room, Dominick grew increasingly more anxious. After a few long rings, the other line finally picked up. "Gavin 'ere. Who's this callin'?"

Dominick froze at the sound of a familiar voice, the tread on his shoes squeaking on Susan's linoleum floor. "Gavin! This is Detective Antonelli. Listen, Dalton is there in Portree. He's the man who sent Giddeon after Ellora. Yes. He's there."

Shuffling through some paperwork that he held in his hands, Dominick finally found the correct one. "Yeah, he bought that old abandoned warehouse a month ago..." Dominick skimmed down the page, "the umm... The Armadale House on Bank Street. Wait, what? Well, where's Ellora? Go get her! She's in danger," Dominick roared into the speaker. "I'm on the next flight out. Stay together." He ended the call, his body rocking with a flood of adrenaline.

Dominick was muttering under his breath in disbelief. "I can't believe he didn't send someone else. Shit. I can't believe I have to fly all the way out there... again. Fuck!" As he was gathering all his belongings, the sight of Susan stopped him dead in his tracks. Her expression looked grave, her complexion having paled. "I'm sorry if I scared you. I hate the idea of leaving you here while I rush out like this. I wanted to see you safely placed, but you'll be in safe hands with people I trust... I will reach out to you when I get back. Shit, I'm sorry it has to be this way."

The detective was by her side in two quick strides, placing a chaste kiss on either cheek. "I have to go, Suzie Q." Reaching into his back pocket, Dominick retrieved his card and placed it gently into the palm of her hand. "If you need me for any reason or don't feel right about... something, don't second guess yourself. Call me. I will come, I promise." With one more longing glance, he rushed out the door.

Dominick debated on telling Giddeon, but thought it best he clue him in on his return, instead. As he raced his car through lights, he made his way to Hancock Airport, thinking about what he'd find once he set foot back in Portree. The very idea that Dalton could get his sleazy hands on the girl at any moment had him pressing the accelerator to the floor. "I'm coming, Ellora."

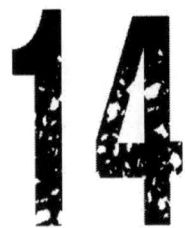

iddeon was surprised when the detective agreed to let him stay at Eva's for dinner. He must be losing his edge because nobody seemed to be worried about this girl's well-being. Either that, or Giddeon was as transparent as water and everyone knew that he couldn't... wouldn't hurt his Angel. That thought had him wondering what that could mean. He'd never cared about anyone. No matter, he was excited to have a hot, homemade meal, and thrilled that he would get to spend some extra alone time with a goddess.

Dominick was headed back over to Dalton's high-rise to talk to Susan some more. He seemed to be anxious to bring down his empire. The man never rested. Giddeon sat back on Eva's overstuffed couch, running his hands through his floppy mess of hair, deep in thought. He hoped the detective could convince the scared girl to cooperate. They needed to find Dalton. *He* needed to find him.

Anger continued to course its way through his veins, causing a prickling sensation to crawl across his skin. The longer Dalton remained unfound, the more anxious Giddeon was to get his hands on him, to finally put an end to all this.

A black cat hopped onto the couch, bringing Giddeon back to his present surroundings. The cat glared at him, his tail twitching in annoyance. "I don't think your cat likes me very much, Angel."

Walking in the room from the kitchen wearing an amused smile, Eva approached her lounging visitor with a loaded wooden spoon. "D.K. is used to being king of this castle. Plus, he's claimed that couch you're camped out in as his throne." She laughed loud and hard when she observed the stare-off between the two dark males.

"Here, try this." Eva crouched low, bringing the hot spoon to his salivating mouth.

"This smells fucking fantastic." Leaning forward, Giddeon slurped down the scalding hot bite, groaning loudly as the food traveled down his throat and into his empty stomach. "Oh my God. What is this? It's gotta be the best tasting thing I've ever had!"

Eva wore a proud smile as she retracted the spoon from his lips before he took a bite out of her utensil. "It's chicken Riggies. I made meatballs to go along with it, and I've got fresh garlic bread baking in the oven. My Grammy showed me how to make this. It's a family recipe and my favorite dish."

Closing his eyes, Giddeon savored the smell and reveled in the creamy sauce left behind from his bite. "I'm starved. I hope it's almost ready, now that you teased me with a taste." When he opened his eyes, he had two sets staring back at him. The first belonged to Eva as she gazed down at him with an expression he'd never seen coming from a beautiful woman like her... adoration.

The second belonged to her cat, D.K., who had crawled into his lap. Curiosity got the better of him as he watched the furball pace in circles on his lap before settling in. "What does D.K. stand for?"

Eva's smile grew wide as she sauntered back into her open kitchen. "Why, Dark Knight, of course." She hummed an unknown melody that stirred something deep down inside the pit of his stomach as he zeroed in on her curvaceous hips, which were swaying side to side as she prepared to set the table.

Prying his eyes off her proved to be more difficult than it should've been. He looked down at the curious hairball purring on his lap. "So, Dark Knight, huh? That's a pretty cool name." The slightly suspicious animal hesitated when Giddeon extended a hand to pet him.

"He's a little skittish around strangers. I rescued him from the shelter when I got my first place after I sobered up. He'd been terribly abused by his previous owner. I guess we were both in need of someone."

Giddeon studied the dark cat with an entirely different perspective. "You and me both, buddy." Giddeon took a chance and ran his fingertips through the medium length hair, ignoring the low warning growl. After a minute, D.K. began to relax into his touch. "I understand. You're protective of her and guarded around others, aren't you, buddy? I get it." D.K. stared at him a few more minutes, then nuzzled his head against the proffered hand.

Giddeon wasn't necessarily a cat person, or a people person, either, for that matter, but for some reason, the small trusting gesture got to him... just a little. This previously battered cat had suffered in the past. "I can relate, dude," he whispered to the purring pile of hair seated comfortably up against his stomach.

"C'mon in. Everything is ready."

Hell yeah! Starving, he gently lifted the contented cat up to his face. "Sorry, dude. A guy's gotta eat." D.K. nuzzled his head under his new friend's chin. Giddeon had to admit, he was a pretty cool cat. After placing him down on the warm spot he'd created, Giddeon trotted into the kitchen.

He stopped abruptly as Eva was blocking his path, mouth wide open in shock. "Wow! I can't believe he just did that. D.K. hates guys. Always hisses at them."

Giddeon didn't like the sound of that. "Just how many guys do you bring up here?"

Eva snorted at the question in annoyance. "Friends and family, Giddeon, and it's none of your business anyways."

The dark man looked over at the equally dark cat and smirked. "Good Job, my man. Keep those other assholes away. I like you more already."

Making his way over to the table, and the location of

the purely heavenly aroma, Giddeon spotted a huge, heaping plate piled high with the delicious pasta. Plopping down in his chair, Giddeon grabbed his fork with wide eyes, ready to dive right in. Before he could shovel the food into his big mouth, Eva stopped him. Confused, Giddeon looked to her. She bowed her head with closed eyes and began to say grace. Once again, the woman surprised him.

Giddeon was awed at the words she uttered in prayer. He couldn't keep his eyes off her. She sounded like his mother. She, too, always said grace before every meal. He realized right then and there how much he wanted this woman. He wished he was someone else... anyone else besides the marked up and broken man who sat beside her. Giddeon desperately wanted to hold her in his arms, to kiss and caress every inch of her body. But more than anything else, he desperately wished he could deserve her love... deserve *her*.

Every time Giddeon thought he had a handle on this bold, crass woman, she blew him away with something new. "Eat up! It'll get cold." Eva caught him staring in reverence at her while she was shoveling the pasta into her mouth. Mimicking her, Giddeon started in on his meal, but couldn't help but keep his eyes trained on hers. This beautiful woman impressively annihilated her plate like a savage huntress.

Eva packed her cheeks with her favorite food while her eyes roved over the imposing man darkening the atmosphere in her dining room. She noticed several scars scattered throughout his body. He had been dwelling in hell for so many years. Alone. No wonder his temper and violent nature was so fine tuned. Her heart ached for him. She wanted so much to pull him into her arms and show him what love could feel like.

Her curious nature was getting the better of her. She wanted to know how he got each and every one of them, but decided that she should try to refrain herself... to let him enjoy his hot meal. It was a pleasure long overdue for him.

Giddeon broke the comfortable silence first, pointing his fork at her. "After you left to start over, did you ever go back to see your mother and step-father?"

Eva swallowed hard, forcing a large piece of bread down. "Umm. I did go back a month or two after I'd ran away." Hesitating for a moment, Eva took a large swig of her Pepsi before continuing. "I still loved my mother, despite all she'd done to me. I knew that it was the addiction ruling her personality in those days. When I went back, the house had turned into a full-fledged druggie hang-out. There where people passed out on the floors, and empty bottles and needles littered all over. I ran upstairs, searching for her, and when I found her hunched over the tub filled with vomit in the bathroom, I realized she was beyond my help."

Having lost her appetite, Eva pushed her plate to the side and continued. "I helped clean her up, changed her clothes, and took her across the street to a diner. She was so emaciated. I hardly recognized her. She just sat there in a zombie-like state. Her bones were jutting out, and her skin was ashen grey. She never uttered a word. I fed her like a young child, nursing her back to health. Once she started to come around, I tried to get her to come with me. To get some help. To leave Rob."

Eva brought her hand up to cradle her head. Pinching her eyes closed, she continued. "She grew extremely agitated and violent, just belligerent. We were kicked out of the diner because of her erratic behavior. Once outside, she tried her best to convince me to get high with her. Just one more time."

Eva wrung her hands together nervously, looking anywhere in the room but at Giddeon. After a few cleansing breaths, she continued. "I'm ashamed to admit that I was tempted to go back. The thought of that heavenly euphoric feeling spreading through my system had me wavering. Just being that close to the house was a stronger temptation than I thought it'd be. It took all of my strength and willpower to deny her. She wobbled back to the house, slurring something about needing a 'pick me up fix'. I haven't seen her since."

Giddeon shook his head slowly from side to side as he looked over her with an admiration he'd never had toward anyone before. "You're an incredibly brave and strong woman." Giddeon dropped his fork on his empty plate and dipped his weary head. "I wish I could've known you then. I needed a strong person like you in my life. Your conviction... your willpower, is inspirational." His voice dropped lower, almost to a whisper. "Things would've been different. I would've been different."

Eva couldn't contain herself any more. Even though they were only a foot apart, it was too far away to her. Scooting her chair ever closer, she cupped his chin and gently turned him to face her. "Giddeon, you're a survivor. You're a fighter. As your name suggests, you're my mighty warrior. I don't know a single person who could've survived what you have."

Too tired to argue, he simply stated, "Look at me, Eva. I'm a mess. If you only knew the things I've done... you'd run from me screaming." When Eva shook her head to argue, he interrupted her sternly. "You should run. I'm a dangerous disaster, barely holding myself together." The energy between the couple sparked something intense inside of them, igniting a flame that grew the longer they gazed at one another.

Deciding after a few breathless moments later to change the subject, Eva ran her fingers over the white circular scar tissue sporadically scattered over his arms, trying desperately to be hidden underneath his elaborate tattoos. "What are these from?"

As if forgetting their presence, Giddeon lifted a curious brow and looked down at the hand gently stroking the sensitive tissue. Her delicate touch sent chills up his spine, spurring his body to life. He ached to feel her body pressed against the source of his desire. His eyes drifted closed for a few beats of his accelerated heart at her tenderness.

Seeing his reaction, Eva continued the feather-light circular motions. Every passing second that her fingers continued to caress his skin had heightened his desire to take her. Goosebumps raised his heated flesh, arousing parts of him that had been unaffected for a long time. Giddeon fought against himself to not hiss at her suggestive ministrations.

If she continued to caress him like that, he would tell her anything she wanted to know. He was putty in her soft hands. All he could think of at that moment was pouncing on her, peeling off all her clothes, layer by layer, and kissing a path down her sinfully curvaceous body. The latter seemed to be a much more desirable idea.

Before he knew it, his lips parted and he started revealing the story against his will. He fought control of his own mind as visions of Eva undressing for him danced through his head. The raw need to feel her skin against his was becoming overwhelming.

"This was one of many punishments I received while in my second foster family. My foster dad had left the basement door unlocked one day, a room I wasn't allowed in. Curiosity and sheer boredom got the better of me. I walked through the side door located in the kitchen and snuck down the withered, old, creaky stairs and into the damp, musty smelling room. When I turned on the light switch, I was ecstatic at what my eyes found. He had a huge prize shelf of antique model cars." A smirk inched its way onto Giddeon's face as he recalled the memory.

Eva couldn't help but smile, thinking of a handsome young Giddeon drooling over shiny model cars. "I was helplessly drawn to them. The artfully crafted models, bright spectacular paint, and shiny chrome wheels drew me like a moth to a flame. My father and I used to put model cars, just like them, together, then played around with them when we were finished."

Giddeon ran his strong hands through his messy locks, then leaned his elbow on the kitchen table. "This one model in particular, I swear to God, was an exact replica of one I had built. Before I could stop myself, I found myself climbing up the metal shelving like a ladder to the top to grab it. The candy apple red GT Shelby 500 was silently begging me to pick it up, to play with it... to appreciate it. Just as I had grasped it, my drunk foster father stormed into the room with a bottle of gin in hand and a murderous glare directed hatefully at me.

"His clumsy thunderous approach startled me. I knocked the model car onto the concrete floor, and watched in horror as it crashed to the floor in slow motion and smashed into a million tiny pieces. I should've been more scared for my own safety, but I was devastated over the broken memory. Damaged. Unfixable. And ruined, just like me." Eva's heart broke for the young boy.

"His face turned about four different shades of red and purple as he gritted his teeth and clenched his fists, readying himself to come at me. He tore me off the shelving by my hair and dragged me down to the cold concrete floor. I remember feeling the remnants of the broken model pieces digging into my back. I lay still, waiting for the punishment to come, watching as he slowly took the cigarette that dangled precariously out of his mouth. He lowered it to my chest and pressed down, burning me. I still remember the smell of my own flesh burning.

"I know he wanted the satisfaction of hearing me scream and cry in pain, or for me to put up some sort of a fight. I gave him none of that. I didn't move. I never made a sound. I just watched him. His anger grew as he burnt me over and over, until finally, he pressed it so hard, he put the cigarette out on me. I just smiled at him. I could see in his eyes that I really freaked him out. He tried to hide it, but I could see the fear in his eyes as he looked at me. When I started laughing in triumph, he removed his belt and beat me unconscious with it."

Eva let out a devastated sigh. It was a very unnatural sound coming from such a strong woman. Guilt welled up inside Giddeon; he felt like an asshole for telling this story when they were having such a good evening. What the fuck was wrong with him? "Oh, Eva. I'm sorry. I shouldn't have told this story. I ruined a good dinner."

Leaning down, the golden-haired Angel placed delicate kisses on every scar in sight. The wet sensation of her tender lips on his skin ignited something between them. He froze on the spot.

"Don't you dare be sorry, Giddeon. Don't you EVER apologize to me. None of this is your fault. I asked you to tell me. I just can't imagine someone who was paid to look after you, by the state for fuck's sake, would do this to a young child. I can't even imagine what you went through while stuck in that house. My heart breaks for what you've been through, the cruelty you faced. Knowing that you were forced to sleep under the same roof as those monsters..."

Giddeon dragged a rough fingertip against her plump lips, silencing her. When he was sure his stubborn Angel would stay quiet, he removed his finger and thumbed away the traitorous tears that snuck out. "Don't you cry for me, Eva. I looked forward to every single strike. It's the only way I could feel anything at all anymore. I walked around in a fog, a sort of haze that kept me from reality for so long that I became numb to the world around me, drowning in my own guilt and despair.

"Pain forced me to feel. It has been the one and only thing that made me feel like a living breathing human being again. I'm not worth a single one of your tears. I'm a monster." Giddeon was breaking. Too much raw pain was crashing to the forefront. Bowing his head, he once again fought the tears that burned the back of his eyes and cooled a path down his cheeks.

The anniversary of his parents' murders, and the knowledge of who'd been behind it all along, was too much for him. Before he could stop himself, he was cast back into a memory he ached to forget.

The petrified boy stood in the same spot he'd been left in for several hours, still clutching the dagger. His mind had been frozen in time. Like a movie stuck on pause, he was unable to cope with the horror that had taken place right in front of him.

An alarming, earsplitting horn blared obnoxiously just outside of the opened window, breaking up the eerie silence in the room. The deafening blast startled the boy as he flinched and blinked back to his devastating reality. All his limbs and joints were numb from lack of movement for so long.

Robotically, he finally forced his eyes down. His mommy and daddy lay slumped over on the ground. He stared for a long time... waiting for them to move.

They didn't.

Little Giddeon crept carefully over to their still forms and saw them bleeding. A LOT. Tears spilled out as the scared boy cried out and dashed the rest of the way to their sides. When his bare feet hit the pool of blood, he slipped, falling hard to his knees. He skidded across the cold crimson puddle on the tiled floor.

Wrapping his arms around her cold form, the boy tried to wake her. "Mommy, it's me. Wake up. They're gone now,

Mommy. It's going to be okay now." The small boy zeroed in on the grotesque wound across her neck. Tears streamed down his cold cheeks. Frantically whipping his head from side to side, he searched around himself for something that could help her.

Little Giddeon grabbed his favorite superman cereal bowl that had fallen from the overturned table, and began scooping up the cold, goopy blood on the floor. Lifting up the full bowl, he tried his best to pour it back in the gaping hole. "I'll put it back, Mommy. You'll be okay. I'll put it back." He continued to scoop and pour, trying helplessly to put her back together. Finally looking over to his daddy's frozen form, he shouted, "Daddy, wake up! Mommy's hurt! Help her, Daddy!" He continued to shout at him as he shook his stiff body frantically. "Oh, Daddy, you're cold, too." Getting an idea, Giddeon jumped up and ran to his room. He raced back as fast as he could, determined to revive them.

"I'm back. You're so cold. Here... I've got my Ironman blankie." Little Giddeon remembered his dad telling him it had special powers and would protect him when he was scared. He spread the blankie over their stone figures.

The boy stood... waiting. As he stared down at them, he realized it was all his fault.

He just stood there. He didn't help Dad fight the monsters, or stop his mommy from walking in when the scary, angry men were yelling. He just hid there and didn't do anything. If his mommy had his blankie, it would've protected her. Instead, he let the monsters come and hurt his mommy and *daddy.*

Now, they were in heaven… together. Giddeon wanted to be in heaven with them.

He thought that maybe if he laid down beside them long enough, God would take him, too. Giddeon was scared and didn't want to be all alone. What if those monsters came back for him? Giddeon crawled under the worn, faded blanket and laid down between both his parents. He desperately wanted his mother to wrap him up in her protective arms and tell him everything would be okay. He snuggled next to her cold, hard side and wrapped his trembling arms around her. "I love you, Mommy."

But, he knew nothing would be okay. Not after that day. Not ever again.

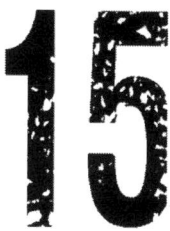

Giddeon came around a while later to the sensation of Eva running her hands up and down his arms softly. Once his eyes focused, he gazed directly into her watery, bright blue eyes. Every time she made contact with his skin, she brought him out of his perpetual hell and back into the world around him. She had power over his darkness. She had power over the beast that laid claim over him.

He wasn't sure how much time had passed, but he was no longer at the kitchen table. Giddeon was hunched over his knees on her couch. Eva knelt down beside him, sobbing quietly. A sick feeling coursed through him. Had he revealed that memory out loud? His strong Angel gently laid her head on his knees, her arms draped over his lap.

The emotionally raw man ran his hands through his messy locks, hating that he lost control and blacked out right in front of her. Bitterness found its way back into his heart, hardening it once again. A cold front iced over any lingering emotions that tried to come to the surface. Desperately needing some air, Giddeon pushed Eva off of him and away.

His hardened expression looked down at the only person brave enough to actually *want* to be around him. Surprisingly enough, she didn't seem hurt by his sudden coldness. Instead, she glared at him with fierce determination.

"Don't," Eva forced out through clenched teeth. She was on her feet in an instant. "Giddeon, you can *try* to push me away and shut me out all you want, but I'm not so easily dismissed or chased away. Not even you can break my strong will. Whether you like it or not, I'm here, and I'll always be here. Right by your side." Eva approached the agitated man teetering so close to the edge, ignoring his warning glances.

Placing her hands on her hips in a defensive stance, she continued in a low, stern voice. "Through it all... the good, the bad, and the terrifying, I will *not* be chased away, so you'd better get used to having me around."

Giddeon pushed through her stance abruptly, shaking his head as he walked away. Eva ran after the retreating man. There was no way in hell she was letting him leave like this, not after all that had happened, and definitely not after all he'd revealed to her. After the story he told while in a trance-like state, Eva's heart ripped wide open. She decided right then and there she wasn't going to fight it anymore. She tried with all her might to stay on the straight and narrow, but all her efforts to be his counsellor, and *only* his counsellor, had failed. She was falling for this tortured soul, and it was tearing her apart inside.

He had been pushed away, discarded, and abused his whole life. He needed someone who could love him, a constant in the midst of all his chaos. More than anything, he needed someone to *stay*. No matter what.

Giddeon stopped short a few feet from the front door, turning on his heel to face Eva. He didn't want to be cruel to the one and only person to act as though they really cared what happened to him. She deserved better. The momentum of Eva's haste to catch up to her dark warrior had her crashing into his chest.

His cold, rigid arms instinctively wrapped around his Angel to prevent her from falling. Blowing out a steadying breath, Eva slowly ran her hands up his broad chest. The adoring, determined look in her eyes knocked the wind out of him, catching him completely off guard.

It was an expression he hadn't seen from her, and she was directing it right at him. Giddeon's body stirred. Emotions he'd never had for a woman before awoke all his senses. Lust. Need. Wanting. The overload of feelings to his system caused his whole body to quake under her tender touch.

His body grew warm, reacting to his beautiful Angel as she ran her hands over his shoulders and into his thick hair. His heart awoke, slamming hard into his chest, when a jolt of adrenaline coursed through every limb and extremity. When she tugged on a fistful of hair, his body became hyperaware of the erotic beauty standing before him.

All of a sudden, every nerve in his body was alive, awakened to everything around him, including the lust-filled wanting in her hooded eyes that mirrored his own desperate need. He noticed the way her golden hair shimmered under the harsh florescence of the entryway light, and the feel of her soft, creamy skin, clear of any makeup, as he ran his fingertips over her cheek.

She grabbed hold, pulling him in tighter, and her intoxicating scent accelerated his heart like a powerful aphrodisiac. Giddeon shivered as her heavy breaths fanned over his face. He closed his eyes briefly as Eva ran her fingernails into his scalp, taking him to heights he'd never experienced before.

He desperately wanted her. Even if it was just one night, Giddeon wanted to give his Angel everything he had left to give.

This woman was weakening him. He could feel the last bit of control slipping away. She had this incredible power over him. Whenever Eva was around, Giddeon no longer suffered from the overbearing pull that the beast had over him, keeping him a prisoner in the darkness. When she was near, that part of him remained quiet and hidden.

His dark eyes shot open when her hot wet lips kissed a path up his neck, rousing him back to the present. "Eva," he groaned out. Against his body's wishes, he tried one last time to push her away with the last reserves of strength he had. "Don't. You don't want this. You deserve better than a disgusting piece of shit like me."

Eva shook her head in defiance, her lips dragging against his neck at the action, and gave his neck a little bite. Giddeon shuddered, a gritty groan elicited from deep within.

"You can't get rid of me, Giddeon. I have made my choice. I will stand by you. I will be there with you in your darkest moments." She placed several more kisses up his neck then continued. "I will be with you through it all." She continued her soft kisses down his neck and across his collarbone, smiling against his skin when he hissed out a breath.

Giddeon pulled Eva away again, this time holding her at bay. He didn't want this Angel to be exposed to his demons. He didn't want her to see him at his worst. He didn't want to drag her down into his hell. She deserved to be put up on a pedestal. He wanted her so bad, but knew she deserved better. With sad eyes, he proclaimed brokenly, "You can't change me, Eva."

The strong-willed girl jumped up to defend her actions. "I'm not trying to change you, Giddeon. I'm simply trying to help you walk a path that will eventually lead you to hope for a better life. For happiness."

His heart constricted at the pleading look in her eyes and the conviction in her voice as she looked deep inside him. "That's not what I meant, Angel." His voice dropped to a soft gravel. "You don't understand. I died right there with them that day." He pointed to his heart. "This is dead. I've suffered nothing but loss and pain for so long, I don't think I'm capable of loving someone like you the way you deserve to be loved. I know I'm not worthy of having someone like you love me. I can't give anything back. The only things residing in me anymore is hatred, vengeance, bitterness, and guilt. My demons leave no room for anything else."

When Eva shook her head, Giddeon captured her chin in his rough hands. "I'm not the man you want me to be, Eva. I never will be. I can't make you happy, and that's what you deserve—a strong man to take care of you, to make all your dreams come true. That man will never be me."

Giddeon let go of her and ran his hands through his dark hair, dipping his head. He was pissed at himself for saying all that shit when he wanted nothing more than a night of passion with his Angel. But everything he said was true. And he fucking hated himself for it. When he looked up at Eva through his lashes, he was shocked to see her shaking in anger.

Without warning, Eva pushed Giddeon hard in the chest. A jolt of electricity sparked at the point of contact, waking other parts of his long dead body. She was seething in anger, and it was adorable.

"Who the hell ever said I wanted, or needed, a knight in shining armor? What gave you the impression that I'm looking for someone to take care of me? I've taken care of myself all my life. I'm not some weak chick who needs a man to fucking hold my hand through life. I can take care of myself! Always have!"

Eva pushed Giddeon harder this time, and he looked down on her condescendingly and smiled, egging her on. Grabbing fistfuls of his shirt, the pissed off blonde pushed Giddeon hard up against the wall, knocking down keys that hung on a loop by the door. Giddeon raised a challenging brow and a crooked smirk, awaiting the next outburst from his Angel. He was again caught off guard as she attacked his mouth instead, crashing her lips to his.

Her fervent aggression sparked a hungry need deep inside of him that grew with each move of her punishing lips on his. Having lost all power to push her away, Giddeon reciprocated. Their lips crashed together in a desperate frenzy to devour one another. Eva dominantly sucked on his bottom lip, biting down, while curling her fingers into his hair and pulling down hard, roughly positioning his head where she wanted it. Giddeon groaned euphorically as the mixture of pleasure and pain shook him to the core. Burning electric currents coursed through his body, pulsating in the pit of his stomach then rippling outward. Eva's tongue dipped in and out of his waiting mouth, erotically massaging it in a manic rhythm that quickly became his undoing.

Giddeon wrapped his arms around her delicate body

tightly, his fingers gripping her hips with almost painful pressure as he brought her body closer. He needed her closer. A deep growl left his heaving chest as an unfamiliar dark desire clawed its way to the surface. Feeling her pelvis grind suggestively against him pushed him right over the edge. He wouldn't be able to control himself much longer. Her punishing tongue was driving him mad; any more of this and he would take her… right there against the wall.

Her throaty promise was finally his undoing. "I'm going to pour out all my love and devotion onto you. You don't have to give anything back. Let me love you, Giddeon. Let me show you what that feels like. You don't have to do anything. Just accept it." His golden Angel cupped his face and brought her plump, swollen lips back to his, slowing the kiss down. She brushed her hot tongue along the seam of his lips in a provocative torture that almost brought him to his knees.

The marked man was a goner. He couldn't fight her any longer. Giddeon opened up to her, ready and willing to take her in his mouth. She didn't disappoint. His Angel tasted of sweet honey. Eva let out tiny breathless moans as Giddeon took control of the kiss. The noise awoke a carnal desire inside of him. He spun them around, crashing her tiny frame into the wall, and extended her hands high above her head, trapping her. Giddeon aggressively deepened the kiss, probing his tongue in and out of her hot mouth in an erotic rhythm that brought them both to frantic heights.

Giddeon's body tremored and quaked with his need to feel her soft skin against his. Muscles coiled and twitched with desperation to take his Angel. Giddeon hadn't experienced so many sensations all at once like this, *ever*. Now that he had been taken over by it, he wanted more. The marked man was becoming addicted to how Eva made him feel when he was with her.

"I want to feel all of you, Eva. I need you. Right now." Eva continued to kiss him in between each breathless word proclaimed. Without hesitation, she tugged his shirt up over his head and tossed it away. He hissed through gritted teeth when the bold girl ran her hands up his tense and twitching ab muscles and over his chest, her touch leaving a hot trail behind. The path they took raised goosebumps on his dark, heated flesh.

Giddeon let loose a groan, feeling a different kind of torture that he wasn't used to. The pleasure of each touch and stroke from his Angel was a delicious kind of agony that made him want to beg for more. Pressing all his weight into her as he ground his hips alerting her of his growing need, he managed to growl through tightly gritted teeth, "Bedroom. Now," in between punishing kisses.

Without answering, Eva pushed him across the room, managing to navigate without needing to look. She wrapped her arms around his neck, pulling him in tighter as they stumbled down the hall, half aware of their surroundings. Giddeon gripped the hem of her t-shirt and pulled it over her head in one swift movement, reveling in the sight of her golden hair tumbling down around her lace-covered breasts.

Her chest heaved as she breathed heavily in and out. She gazed at her dark warrior through hooded eyes, ready to give herself to him. Giddeon froze in place, mesmerized by her beauty. She was perfect to him in every way. When he hesitated, Eva took hold of his hand and placed it over her heart.

"If your heart is dead, I'll give you mine." Her words struck the concrete wall that guarded his dead heart and shattered it. He could feel the force of it like a solid punch to the chest.

Giddeon shivered at all the new and unfamiliar emotions that rushed forward, leaving him trembling in her arms. Cupping his Angel's face, he gazed down on her with an adoration and longing he'd never in his life awarded to another person, until Eva. Slowly dipping his head, he captured her lips with his and kissed her with all the feelings coursing through him. He held nothing back. He worshiped her mouth, taking his time to explore her with all the attention she deserved.

Fumbling blindly, he finally found the knob of the bedroom door they were standing in front of. Giddeon wanted to make sure his lips properly worshiped every inch of her perfect body, and he'd need lots of time and space to do so. Eva began unbuttoning his jeans as she nibbled on the delicate skin of his earlobe. She whispered softly, promising, "It's just you and me tonight, Giddeon."

That was it. He pushed past the door with Eva wrapped around him. "Your voice chases away all my demons. With one touch, you bring me out of the darkness and into the light with you." Giddeon gently bent her backwards onto the bed, proclaiming as he kicked the door closed behind them. "You are *MINE* now, Angel."

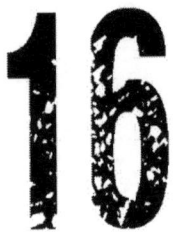

16

Dalton paced the room he'd been holed up in for the last few hours. The longer he waited to be in a room alone with Ellora, the more agitated and reckless he'd become. The stunt he pulled in Ellora's room was an unnecessary risk and a very close call. Gritting his teeth, he pinched his eyes closed, imagining the feel of her soft lips pressed against his.

He couldn't wait any longer. He took it upon himself to up the ante. Desperate times called for desperate measures, after all. His pocket buzzed, signaling an incoming call. Pulling out his cell, he bit out, "Dalton Ramsey Claiborne here."

The man at the other end answered, "Yes, sir. It's done. I did all that you've asked."

Dalton let out an appreciative sigh of relief. "Exemplary work. Now, we wait until he leaves to make my move. I've wired your fee directly to you. Our business is finished here."

"Thank you, Mr. Claiborne, sir. This was most generous of you."

Dalton hung up on the man without as much as a

salutation. Stalking back over to the monitors, he searched for the object of his growing desire. She was working up quite a sweat today. He stared at her for an extremely long time, imagining her petite body writhing on top of his, working up an identical sweat.

His twisted heart accelerated when he thought of her. The time for action was drawing closer. His entire being grew anxious to take her and use her in every way he'd ever dreamed up. Dalton was borderline manic, desperately needing to claim Ellora as his. His plan had to work, and fast. His time was running out where her innocence was concerned. He feared that the large man always around her might possibly beat him to the punch if he waited any longer.

If that bastard took his dark beauty… if he ruined her, Dalton would have no choice but to end them both. After all, he always won, no matter what. They wouldn't have a happily ever after, not while he had a breath left in his body. "Soon enough, darling, I will have you all to myself. There will be no one else standing in the way of our destiny."

He kissed his cleanly manicured fingers and stroked them over her face on the gritty monitor. He zoomed in as she smiled at her friends. This girl… this one little girl held a lot of unrealized power in her hands. She just had to beckon to him, and he'd gladly give up billion dollar deals to be by her side. Hell, he'd already done just that. She had but to ask, and he'd give her the world on a platinum platter.

All his privileged life, Dalton only cared about money, power, and success. He didn't care who he had to destroy along the way. But this raven-haired enchantress barged into his ruthless world and knocked him sideways. His entire empire was now in danger of falling down around him from his silence, the amount he'd spent on his plan to get her back, and his lengthy absence from the company.

He knew that backstabbing prick he hired, Detective Antonelli, was gunning for him, and he wouldn't stop until he had his man. But no one could take him down. He'd made sure of that. He had more men lined up, ready and willing to put everything on the line, to do as he ordered with the snap of his fingers.

Money could always be earned. Loss could always be recovered. But Ellora was the once in a life time opportunity that he simply couldn't... *wouldn't* pass up. Ever.

She'd learn to love him. She'd have no other choice.

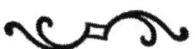

Ellora looked over at Adelle and couldn't help but laugh at her beautiful friend. She was even flawlessly stunning in paint-stained overalls and with plaster stuck in her hair. She practically painted with her pinky up. She was adorable. As always, they broke up into pairs: Behr and Ellora on one side of the warehouse wall, and Gavin and Adelle on the other.

Adelle was wearing an adorable pout as she was

forced by everyone to lend a helping hand. She really despised manual labor. Gavin was all too willing to help instruct her on her terrible painting techniques whenever he could. Like a jackal ready to pounce, he looked forward to every opportunity that became available to get closer to her.

Ellora was indebted to her thoughtful friend for digging up old photos from Kristy of the hardware store when her father had worked there. Her plan was to try to restore it as close to how he had it all those years ago. So, they were painting the newly installed walls a rich, dark burnt orange color, which warmed up the atmosphere of its warehouse coldness. It provided a down to earth, homey feel for the place. She fell in love with it.

Luckily, the painting job was an easy one compared to the pub. Three of the walls were a long, blank uninterrupted expanse. Only the front of the warehouse had large bay windows with large double doors in the center. They could easily kill the painting job in one day. After another hour or so, they stopped for lunch.

Kristy stopped by with two bags filled with food. The woman was a saint. They all congregated at the now polished front counter to stuff their starving bellies. As always, Behr prepared Ellora's plate first, and even laid a cloth napkin on her lap as he kissed her nose. Ellora looked up at this magnificent man adoringly, mouthing, "I love you. So much."

Murmuring softly in her ear, he responded, "And I,

you." His affectionate pale blue eyes and brilliant smile left her spellbound. *Oh, Behr.*

Adelle hopped up onto the counter, refusing to sit on the dusty ground, with her plate in hand. Gavin piled food high onto his plate and sidled up next to her. His eyes roved over the regal beauty from the top of her strawberry colored head and slowly travelled their way down every curve her body boasted, to the soles of her feet. His expression changed from its usually light-humored cocky air, to a profound longing.

When Adelle finally looked to her side and met his eyes, they shared a prolonged unspoken connection, as if they were the only two people in the room. The air was thick with their mutual tension.

Ellora watched them carefully. If she wasn't mistaken, she could've sworn she witnessed sparks flying between them over the past few weeks. Gavin absolutely adored her; he didn't even try to hide it. It pained Ellora to witness their heated and playful flirtations, but neither one ever followed through with their actions and confessed how they truly cared for each other.

Ellora smiled as she watched Gavin snatch away Adelle's plate. Her friend pouted at first, until Gavin arched a knowing brow and asked, "Would my queen like her king to feed her? They're not bloody fingers this time." They both laughed at their obvious inside joke, and Adelle's eyes lit up as she seemed to slip into a daydream and stared into

Gavin's eyes. In their moment, no one else existed... it was just the two of them. Ellora made a mental note to ask her about the bloody fingers joke later.

"So, Adelle, you start teaching here pretty soon, right? Are you excited?" Ellora asked, changing the subject as the air around them was getting much too thick to breathe. Not to mention, the both of them had a terrible habit of interrupting every time she and Behr had a private moment. Tit for Tat.

Adelle answered even as her doe eyes continued to gaze deep into Gavin's. "Aye, that I am. I've always loved school. Now, I've found a way to be in one all the time, and they'll pay me to do it. Nothin' in the world is a better fit for me. I start a week shy of a month from now. I cannae believe it. I'll be in charge of my very own classroom."

Gavin smiled brilliantly at the object of his unspoken desire, loving how her eyes twinkled with excitement as she expressed her joy. When she smiled back at him, he could've sworn his heart skipped a beat then halted altogether. Adelle always managed to steal his breath away. Unable to stop himself, as usual, he reached out to the strawberry ringlet that beckoned to him and twirled it around his paint-stained finger. "I'm so proud of you, lass. I always knew you were somethin' special."

Adelle's porcelain skin blushed pink. Suddenly shy, she looked down at her hands, avoiding his eyes. Gavin placed a finger under her chin, lifting her head up so she was once again looking him in the eyes. "No matter what you may think of me, I always knew you were someone special, and had no doubt in the world that you'd find success in your life."

Ellora could've sworn he whispered, "I only pray that one day you will allow me the honor of being a part of it with you," in a low tone by her ear. As he sealed his proclaimed statement with a tender kiss on her forehead, her heart swelled for them. Something was definitely developing between the two; their chemistry grew with each passing day since Adelle came back from college.

For once, Behr and Ellora got to sit back and watch someone else's intimate moment. She looked up to her large protector, and he mouthed the words, "I love you, Lor." His large frame bent down to place a loving kiss on her soft lips, then laughed as she still had a mouthful of food packed in her cheeks.

Ellora decided to once again change the subject and lighten the mood from the hot and heavy atmosphere that had been lingering in the warehouse all day. There must have been some sort of hex cast on it, she thought idly. After all, this was the spot where her father fell in love at first sight with her mother. This building seemed to bring couples together. "So, Behr, what does a girl have to do to get a guided tour up the Trotternish Mountains?"

Adelle perked up at the mention. "Oh, we should all go. We can take 'er up the Quaraing trail. Aye, it's beautiful up there, with much to see. We can pack a little picnic and lunch up at the 'table top'. Aye, she'll love that."

Behr's eyes lit up at the suggestion, nodding in agreement. "Aye, love. I did promise ya a hike. That's a promise I intend to keep. It'll do ya some good to take a break from all this back breaking labor and enjoy Skye's wondrous majesty."

Adelle clapped her hands excitedly. "Yay, it's settled then. Let's plan on this upcoming weekend for sure."

Ellora nudged Behr playfully. "It's about time you take me out in public. I was starting to think you were embarrassed to be seen with this Yankee."

Behr dropped his food and crawled the short distance, forcing her to lean back onto her elbows as he stalked over her. Wrapping his large arms tightly around her tiny waist, he drew her closer to him. "Never. I just wanted my handywoman all to myself. I'm of a selfish sort. Now that I 'ave you, I'm never letting you go."

Ellora wrapped her arms around his neck. "I'm not going anywhere without you by my side."

When their lips brushed together shamelessly, a symphony of groans and fake gags effectively broke the spell. Their breath mingled together as they laughed breathlessly at their not so subtle friends. "Ugh, get a room, you two!"

Just to spite her interrupting friend, Ellora decided to teach her a lesson. Tilting her head to the side, she tangled her hands into Behr's dark locks and brought him down to her. She not so gracefully kissed him deeper, as loudly and obnoxiously as possible, even going as far as making indecent slurping noises.

Behr didn't object in any way, playing right along with her all too willingly. "That's right, love. Gobble me right up. 'Ave your fill."

After their grotesquely sweet display, everyone continued eating their lunch. Ellora looked around at her new family, grateful to have them in her life. "All right, I'll take a break from this place and plan on a weekend of adventure. But... until then, I'm going to crack the whip on you and try to get as much work done as possible."

Adelle groaned exasperatedly. "You're the worst boss ever."

Gavin broke his eye contact with Adelle to taunt Ellora. "Ah, lass, keep your bedroom toys at home and save them for this grizzly over here. Aye, he's the one who needs taming." Leaning into his strawberry-haired queen, Gavin whispered not so low in her ear, "Donnae worry, lass. I'll be happy to massage out all the kinks later on... in my room." Adelle slapped him half-heartedly as he wiggled his naughty eyebrows at her.

They finished up with lunch and began cleaning up the empty cartons and containers. At the sound of the newly installed bell chime over the entry way doors, they all looked over to see who the new arrival was. Isaac from Jan's

Hardware store strolled in with some bags in tow. Ellora had called ahead to order some extra screws, finishing nails, spackle, and some painter's tape.

"'Ey there, Ellora. I told Bree I'd just deliver this stuff over, seeing as you're so busy. Wow! This place is really takin' shape." Behr stalked over and snatched the items from him with a hard glare. Ellora mentally shook her head at him. Isaac was still in high school, for crying out loud. But Behr didn't hesitate to show his dominance around other guys who showed the slightest interest in her. This was probably the result of his ex, Shannon, after years of infidelity.

"Thanks, Isaac. I really appreciate that." He circled around, taking in all their progress.

"Aye, the place looks well on 'er way. A contractor business, eh? So, we'll be kinda working together on a lot of projects then, yeah? I mean, Jan's and your business. You should apply for the contractors' benefits card. You'll get outstanding rates and discounts on bulk items."

Ellora laced her fingers with Behr's, easing his mounting tension at Isaac's slip in his word choice. "I'll do that. Thanks, Isaac. You've been a terrific help."

Giving her a salute with his hands as a goodbye, he was halfway to the door before turning on his heel. "By the way, Behr, your parents were in the store earlier today."

Behr grew rigid, freezing on the spot after years of unresolved resentment and anger. "So?" was all he gave as a response. Ellora had never seen this side of him before. The bitterness that came off him was so thick, you could cut it with a knife.

"Yeah, they inquired after you, and when Bree let them know about everything that has happened in recent months, they seemed interested to know all about Miss Ellora. Everyone within earshot sang your praises, of course." Isaac's face reddened at his admission before he continued. "Your mother expressed her desire to meet you and..."

Behr interrupted him before he could finish, pushing him out the door in a shocking display of anger. "A'right, we get the point. Thank you, Isaac, but we 'ave lots of work to do." Slamming the door, he marched over to his forgotten paint roller and picked up where he'd left off.

Ellora looked to Gavin and Adelle for an explanation, but they just shrugged. He was now extremely agitated and muttering incoherent things to himself through clenched teeth. She carefully approached him. Behr was quite intimidating when he was like this. Hearing about his parents had obviously upset him. They had, after all, abandoned him when he was still young. He had just showed everyone that he was far from past it.

"Behr, are you okay?" Her heart constricted when he hadn't even looked her way or acknowledged her presence. It made her stomach churn. "Behr. You're scaring me. Please, don't shut me out. Talk to me."

The seething man hissed out a breath like he'd been slapped. Dropping the roller, he wrapped the petite girl up into his strong arms. "I'm nae mad at you, love. I just cannae believe they ask other townies about my well-being. The cowards! If they really cared at all, they'd come and see for themselves. It riles me so, that they dare ask about you. They donnae have a right to ask. They donnae deserve to know you."

The heavy weight of his confession slammed into Ellora like a punch to the chest. She wanted to wrap her arms around Behr and console him, to relieve him from the unmerciful cruelty his parents bestowed on him so many years ago. No one should have to carry around that much resentment and bitterness.

"Why don't we both go to them? You know, you could introduce me to them, and maybe we could all just sit down and talk. I think enough time has passed. I think the time has come for you to make contact with your parents, Behr."

All too suddenly, he let her go, whipping his hands away, and stepped back as if her words had burned him. Ellora flinched at his reaction, and his booming voice rattled her spine. "Why the Devil should I go to them? I already told you once before that I tried that, only to have my own flesh and blood disown me and slam the door in my face. If they really want to know anything about my life or who's in it, it's best they come 'an ask me. Not the rest o' the Isle."

Behr's face slowly turned about three shades of red.

His powerful jaw ticked in frustration as he ran his large hands through his dark hair. His deep, throaty baritone bounced around the near empty warehouse, vibrating the windows. Ellora's voice came out sounding unsure and hesitant. She didn't want him cross with her, but she couldn't seem to keep her mouth closed or let the subject drop.

"Behr... it's just that..." She nervously fiddled with her fingers. "Well, you never know when your father's time here will be up. I do remember the story you told me. You said his health was failing him. That was so many years ago... years wasted with hurtful feelings of betrayal and bitterness. It might be time to drop that heavy burden. The weight of all that on you is enough to bring the strongest of men down. You're a good man, Behr. Leave the past where it belongs and go see your parents. I wish every single day that I had mine here with me. It hurts my heart, knowing they'll never meet you or see how happy you make me. If you hold on to this bitterness and he passes away, you'll feel the most incredible, debilitating guilt that will tear you apart inside. It will haunt you for the rest of your life." Ellora ran her trembling hands up his arms and cupped his face.

"The regret you feel from it will cripple you... You won't ever be able to take it back. Ever." Behr shook from anger, or out of sheer frustration. She knew him well enough to know how incredibly stubborn he could be. The thought of possibly getting rejected and hurt once more was not something he wanted to experience again. But, at the same time, the realization that flashed over his features of his father's depleting health and ticking timeline was also a harsh reminder that the time for reconciliation was dwindling.

For some reason, Ellora was compelled to rush the reunion. Behr hated to make rash decisions. He liked to sit back and think about all his options. Even though she knew this, Ellora kept talking. "No one is guaranteed a tomorrow."

"STOP!" Behr's sudden shout had the petite girl jumping back and away, startled by his thunderous bellow. Her heart pounded inside her chest as his anger was now directed right at her. "Leave this be, Ellora. It's nae any of your business." He snarled through tightly clenched teeth. Before she could stop herself, tears collected around her shocked eyes and spilled over the side.

Ellora was furious at herself for making him so angry. She could see it was a raw subject for him. Why couldn't she just shut her mouth? The emotionally torn girl wrapped her arms around herself, feeling nauseated, her gut twisting and churning from nerves. "I'm... I'm sorry, Behr." Her whispered voice cracked on his name. His mood and expression changed just as fast as his temper had come.

After a few moments passed, he looked horrified with himself. He never wanted to yell at her. He knew she was right, but he wasn't yet ready to face the man, and acted as though he was being pushed to make a rash decision. He never meant to lash out at the very reason his heart beat. Now, she was crying, trying her best to hold the tears back for his sake. He was such a bastard. "Ellora I...I'm sorry. I've gotta get out of 'ere. I need some fresh air."

Ellora stepped forward, swiping away runaway tears. "Behr, please don't go. I'm sorry. Please... don't be angry with me."

He gave one more sorrowful look at the teary-eyed girl who always took the very breath from his lungs. "I'll be out on the water if ya need me, love." He then stormed out, slamming the door behind him. The crash made everyone jump.

Frozen in the very spot she'd been left standing in, Ellora stared at the door, willing him to come back. How had things escalated so quickly? How had this even started? As time ticked by at a painstakingly slow pace, the devastated girl finally crumpled to the cold floor.

Ellora was moments away from vomiting. Bringing trembling hands up to her face, she silently sobbed right there in the middle of the warehouse floor. The very idea that Behr was so mad at her, that he needed to get away from her... needed air and space, struck her aching heart like it was being carved out with dull knives.

She could feel the overwhelming absence of Behr from her spirit, and it suffocated her. Ellora began to hyperventilate, and struggled with herself to gulp in air. On the verge of a full blown panic attack, Ellora was moments away from falling apart. What if he was done with her? What had she done?

Adelle rushed to her friend's side and crouched down by her side. "Ah, don't you cry, Lor. He was out of line, and he knows it and probably feels terrible."

Gavin knelt down on her other side to comfort her. "Aye. Did ya nae get a look at the 'ol grizzly's face? He is plenty ashamed of himself. I'd wager a bet he'll come running back in here beggin' your forgiveness after some time on the water." Gavin added, smirking down at the shaken girl, "You just witnessed the reason why we call him the Grizzly Bear. Aye, a soft teddy bear he is not. It's best you observed his outburst now, rather than later." Gavin chuckled at his own joke.

Adelle rubbed soothing circles on her back. "Damn the ass. I'll give him a tongue lashing when he gets back here. Donnae worry yourself. You are the very air he breathes. And from what I'm seeing now, you feel the same. Why don't you go to the terminal and rent a speed boat... Go after him. I know that's what you really want to do. Gavin and I will stay behind and clean up here. We'll meet you later at Grady's."

The pair helped the girl to her feet and practically pushed her out the door. "Go! Go make up with him, and be sure to tell me all the details later."

Ellora sprinted down Bank Street toward Grady's. She still had wet paint on her and wanted to quickly change out of the soiled clothes. She was overreacting. She knew that. But, after losing her parents and almost losing Behr, it was all too much for her heart to handle. She didn't like how he'd left, and she wanted to right it immediately. The very separation from him made her soul ache. She had become cold and empty without him around.

The thought pushed her faster, and she raced at a breakneck speed as a sick sense of dread pulled her toward him. The chilly wind whipped her hair back behind her as she ran, ignoring the curious stares from passersby. She needed to get to him.

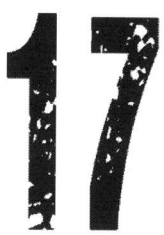

17

ehr wasn't even a few miles out before he turned The Sea Witch around and hit the accelerator. He followed the Trotternish ridge back toward Portree, feeling like such an incredible asshole. A selfish asshole. Too busy complaining about his own parents. Forgetting completely that hers were ripped out of her life. The things he said, he didn't mean. But, surely, the damage had been done, wounding her with his harshness and insensitivity. Behr could still hear what he'd said as it echoed inside his head… and it killed him inside.

Flashes of the hurt confusion in her watery green eyes tore his heart wide open. So much so, that he ran, not knowing what else to do. Now, he had this incredible urgency to get back to her and beg her forgiveness. She was right, after all. Everything she said was right. He'd go to his parents and make peace. He'd be proud to declare that she was his, so long as she'd still have him.

He prayed that his angry outburst didn't frighten her away. His temper didn't come like that often, but his parents had always been an unresolved wound that just wouldn't heal. Behr mentally shook his head. That was a poor excuse and one he didn't plan on making again. She deserved better than that. He vowed never to talk to her like that again. He loved her from the very depth of his soul. She was it for him… he planned on marrying her, hopefully someday in the near future.

A screeching noise tore him away from his thoughts, clanging like heavy metal stressing against its gears. An ear-splitting clanking, and a strange sort of clicking from down below in the engine room, filled Behr with dread. If he could just coast to the terminal, he'd get it checked out.

Sweat collected against his brow at the sound of metal grinding against metal. At this rate, he worried that the odds of making it back were getting slimmer and slimmer by the minute. Thick black smoke began to pour out of the room below, and Behr's heart sank. At that moment, he knew The Sea Witch would go down.

The steering wheel he grasped onto jerked hard to the right, tightening and locking in place. Behr tried with all the strength he could muster to pry the wheel back in place. "What the fuck!" he ground out as he strained unsuccessfully to wrench the steering wheel, but it didn't budge. Not even an inch. The engine screeched with a noise loud enough to crack glass, demanding his attention.

He whipped his head back up just in time to see the Ferry heading right for the rocky cliff walls. Hesitating for a split second, reluctant to abandon his beloved boat and livelihood, he finally made his decision and leapt off the side, just moments before it crashed head on into the punishing Trotternish Ridge.

The sound of the impact thundered all around, even while thrashing around underneath the powerful waves. The sea crashed down onto Behr with brutal force, knocking him around like a weightless ragdoll. He tried with all his strength to surface, but the punishing surf rolled and pushed him down again and again. The unforgiving force dragged him dangerously close to the jagged rocks. The more he struggled to keep clear of them, the more they seemed to reach out to him in a sinister way.

Every time he made it to the surface, he had but a moment to suck in a quick breath before he was hit again by the brutal punch of the unforgiving surf. His lungs burned with the effort to hold his breath and fight exhaustedly to break the surface for more air. After each crushing hit from the sea, waves took turns beating down on him like a game. And all Behr could think about, even then, was Ellora.

He had to make it back to her and let her know how much he loved her.

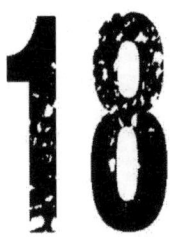

alton lay in wait, a desperate predator on the prowl. The late afternoon shadows kept him hidden as he grew more and more thrilled with overwhelming anticipation, knowing that Ellora was on her way over and he was only moments away from being alone with *his* girl. As time silently ticked by at an agonizing pace, his body quaked with need as he imagined his decadent green-eyed obsession in this very room with him. Finally, after long last, they'd be alone.

This was his chance; one he could hardly wait to take. Dalton's ears perked up at the not so far off sound of boots pounding up the old stairway. His heart swelled and thundered rapidly inside his chest as the footsteps grew closer. "Come to me, my love," Dalton hissed to himself. Moments later, she burst through the door in a rush and kicked it closed behind her with her boot clad foot.

Dalton watched with morbid amusement as she kicked off her ugly manly boots, sending them flying in opposite directions. The frantic girl breezed past the silent intruder, and he inhaled her scent deeply as she went, completely unaware of his dark presence. Dalton frowned as her usually tempting smell was tainted with paint, sawdust, and murky sea air. He despised it. She didn't belong here... with *him*.

Desire quickly morphed to blind anger as he thought of how many times that ape had his hands all over *HIS* Ellora. She had always belonged to him. She just didn't know it yet. But she would... soon enough. Dalton was brought out of his cloud of fury, and watched with fascination as the girl in question peeled off her soiled shirt right in front of him, tossing into a corner hamper.

Rage bubbled up inside him when he spotted, for the first time, the long jagged scar that marked up the soft delicate skin on her back. He would make Giddeon suffer dearly for daring to touch her in such a way. Dalton must have unconsciously crawled out of his hiding place, because he found himself drawing so close to her that he could smell the fresh scent of the clean shirt she pulled over her head.

Dalton slithered closer, need bringing him every step closer to his love. Obviously still unaware of the ominous presence, Ellora collected the soft black river of hair in her hands and pulled it out of the shirt. Dalton's body stirred in response as she tossed it aside. The action sent a swooshing breeze filled with the scent of her lavender shampoo in his direction. Stray strands brushed across his face as he inched closer.

This was a magnificent torture, and too much for him to bear any longer. With gritted teeth and a wandering hand with a mind of its own, the predator reached out, aching to touch her after so much time had passed.

Ellora froze on the spot. Then, just as quickly, she stepped back and turned on her heel, colliding right into Dalton's chest. She gaped with wide eyes in horror as the Devil himself smiled ruthlessly down at her.

His onyx eyes promised vile things as he hissed out, "At long last... You. Are. Mine."

"No."

Ellora blinked several times and chanted inside her head, *This is just a nightmare, Lor. Wake up... wake up... wake up.* She risked a peek through her lashes at the terrifying monster she knew deep down would still be there. He was staring down at her with dead eyes and a gut wrenching sinister smile. With a heaving chest, Ellora pinched her eyes shut once more, willing him to disappear. This had to be a nightmare. There was no way he was standing in her bedroom. This couldn't be real.

All those wishful thoughts evaporated, and reality came crashing down around her, as the Devil himself wrapped his suffocating arms around her. The trembling girl drew in a shaky gasp as his rigid grip tightened. "I've missed you, Ellora Belle Sutherland." The sound of his sleazy voice uttering her full name in such a creepy way had her stomach bottoming out. The way it slowly rolled off his tongue made her want to vomit. "I've dreamed of the day I'd have my dark and delicate beauty all to myself."

Dalton moved forward, forcing the catatonic girl with him, and Ellora stumbled backward on frozen legs. She was paralyzed by the evil hidden behind his all-consuming eyes. She couldn't pry them away, terrified of what would happen next. She wanted to see her fate coming and needed to stand ready for the fight that was sure to come. With tunneled vision, she sensed rather than witnessed his forceful movements around the room, and winced when her back hit the wall.

Still in a state of shock, Ellora repeated a shaky '*no*' over and over, pushing back against the hard, unwavering chest that knocked hard into hers. Shaking her head from side to side, the unblinking girl finally found her voice. "How... how did you get up here?"

Dalton's thin lips stretched over his teeth as his disturbing smirk widened. "What's wrong, sweetheart? Aren't you happy to see me?" Leaning into her pushing hands, he reveled in her growing despair as she desperately tried unsuccessfully to keep him at a distance. Dalton looked down on his trembling girl. His anger that had been simmering just below the surface, burned deep inside of him as he could see in her eyes that she wished *he* were here to save her.

Loosening his tie, Dalton hissed through tightly

clenched teeth, "I've come all this way to retrieve you, and what do I find?" Once loosened, he methodically unfastened the top buttons of his tailored shirt.

Ellora snapped out of her nightmarish haze and pushed back harder. Finding her voice, she shouted out a high pitched, "NO! GET OUT!" Pounding away on his chest with her tiny fists, she frantically tried to get him to step back. Dalton smiled ruthlessly at her weak efforts, grabbing her wrists before she connected with his face. He easily yanked them back behind her, pinning them against the wall.

Dropping his voice to a menacing octave, the malice in the sound raised goosebumps on Ellora's flesh. "I find you throwing yourself into the arms of that brainless Neanderthal like some kind of desperate floosy. He isn't worth the air you breathe." Her body vibrated with renewed fear at her helplessness. Icy chills trickled down her frozen spine as her mind tried to catch up to the danger that stood in front of her. Gritting his teeth in fury at the thought of another man touching her, Dalton marched them deliberately toward the bed, forcefully dragging the panicking girl along with him.

Ellora yanked back hard, trying desperately to break free from his iron-like, unmoving grip. Her joints popped painfully in protest, on the verge of being yanked out of their socket.

"Haven't I told you once before? It doesn't matter how

far you go, how long you hide, or how much it costs me... I'll always find you. You. Are. *MINE.*" Tapping into her growing panic and adrenaline, the petite girl struggled against the evil that ensnared her. Kicking and bucking, she wildly tried to fight him off of her, but Dalton's grip was unyielding.

"I've been watching you all along, and I know that you're still pure. That beast wasn't man enough to take you, and I won't stand by and watch him touch what belongs to me," Dalton grated out through clenched teeth as he bent the struggling girl onto the bed.

Sweat beaded along her forehead, and her face reddened, the veins in her neck protruding as she huffed and groaned, trying uselessly to escape him. She used every ounce of strength she had to push him off.

Loving the sight of his girl powerless beneath him, Dalton's eyes dilated as they zeroed in on the tiny trickles of sweat that rolled down her temple. Groaning as he leaned down, his tongue darted out, capturing one salty bead, and continued to drag his tongue up the side of her face. Closing his eyes, Dalton savored the salty taste of her struggles. "Ah, yes, my love, I love the unmistakable flavor of your fear."

A blood curdling scream ripped through her chest at his contact. The overpowering man shifted his weight on her, shielding his ear from the astonishingly loud shrieking. This gave Ellora the room she needed, and she brought her knee up hard, connecting with his groin. Dalton went rigid over her, groaning out his pain.

Not satisfied with the first hit, Ellora continued to kick and knee him wildly, hitting every mark she aimed for. His thighs, groin, and stomach all fell victim to her punishing blows. Unable to stop her once she started, Dalton loosened his grip on her arms. Yanking them free, she brought her elbow down hard, cracking him square in the jaw, and continued to rain down punches. The tight space made her hits ineffective against the determination of the now enraged man looming over her.

"I will not strike your face, my love, but it is not wise to anger me. I didn't want to take you roughly, but I will if you make me." Mustering up all her strength, she let loose one more powerful blow, connecting with his teeth and splitting her knuckles wide opened. They both cried out in pain as Dalton raised both hands to his mouth, instinctively checking his face. Ellora ignored her throbbing hands and unleashed a vicious attack with her fingernails, clawing his face savagely.

Taking advantage of the brief moment of space he gave her as Dalton rolled to avoid her onslaught, she rolled to her left, breaking free of him. She called on the last reserves of strength and sprinted for the door. All hope of escape shattered the moment his arms snaked around her waist and tackled her to the ground.

Ellora struggled to crawl away face down, trying with all her might to buck his heavy weight off her. Wooden splinters embedded themselves underneath her nailbeds as she gripped and clawed at the floor in an attempt to gain the upper hand.

With a tone all too calm, Dalton cooed in her ear, "This is not at all how I pictured our first time would go." A crippling dread weighed heavily down on her as the realization of what was to come crashed through her consciousness. Ellora was paralyzed by fear when the clinking sound of his belt unfastening assaulted her ears.

The sound was a deafening ominous threat that pulled her deeper and deeper into despair and had her close to passing out. "The bed would have been a more suitable place for your first time, but this is obviously how you want it. You've made your choice." Tossing the belt aside and unbuttoning his pants, he hissed in her ear, "You want me to just take it... don't you? Well, I'm more than happy to comply with your wish, Miss Sutherland."

Ellora continued to struggle, her screams muffled as he grabbed hold of her hair and pressed her face to the ground. Her tears pooled on the floor beneath her, and bile threatened to spill when he drove his hips down on her suggestively. Ellora's voice, now hoarse, sounded scratchy as she cried out in hysteria. "Dalton, DON'T! Don't do this! Please, Dalton, I'll go back with you, just don't do this. Let me go!" She cringed, repulsed as he brushed his lips over her sensitive earlobe.

"Aaah, yes, there's nothing in this world more beautiful than the sound your voice makes when you beg me."

Tears streamed down her face as the helplessness of her situation washed over her in this impossible position. Small whimpers slipped past her lips before she could stop herself. Ellora didn't want to give him the satisfaction of seeing her fear, but she couldn't help it. She was paralyzed by it. This couldn't happen. Not like this.

"I love hearing my name roll off your tongue in that way. It drives me unbelievably wild." Ellora's eyes widened, and her skin went cold and clammy as all the blood drained from her limbs at the sound of his zipper dragging down the track.

Ellora fought against his weight with renewed vehemence, trying frantically to drag herself toward the door. Carrying both their body weight made this task impossible in her face down position.

Dalton fought against a struggle of his own—Ellora's skinny jeans. He yanked hard, trying to pull the unyielding fabric down. The skin-tight pants were much too tight to pry down while she lay heavily on the buttons in the front. Losing his patience, the determined man growled in frustration as he continued to tug roughly with one hand, while the other pushed her head down to keep her in place.

Hope blossomed inside of the helpless girl when Adelle's loud voice and bouncing form burst through the door, not bothering to knock, like she always did. She was entirely out of breath, as if she'd been running, when she huffed out, "Ellora, you'll never believe who just called... Oh! ELLORA!" Without hesitation, Adelle rushed the stranger straddling her friend. She roughly pulled at his sweat drenched, slicked back hair, yanking and tearing at his blonde locks like a rabid wild animal, screaming the entire time.

"Get off her, you bastard! Help! UP HERE! HELP!" Adelle continued to scream manically as her assault on the terrifying intruder intensified. She slapped and scratched him until he let go of Ellora and turned the full force of his fury on her. Blocking one more slap with his forearm, Dalton raised his fist and backhanded her hard across her cheek, then brought the same hand back around, catching her on the temple and knocking her backwards.

Ellora panicked, frightened for her friend, as he unleashed his fury on her. "No! Dalton! Don't you dare touch her! Adelle, run! Just get yourself out of here!" Ellora was terrified for her, knowing that if Dalton got his hands on Adelle, he wouldn't stop. He was capable of so much evil. Without another look back, Adelle stumbled up and out of the room. Dalton turned his attention back on the object of his twisted desire.

"This doesn't leave us much time." With one more forceful tug, Dalton ripped her jeans mid-way down her thighs with bruising force. Belting out an ear-piercing scream, Ellora forced the noise out of her lungs with a force that could break glass... and didn't stop. The horrifying fear of what was about to happen, and the lack of air, clouded her vision, drawing her closer and closer to blacking out.

Fighting the pull, Ellora caught glimpse of a silhouette of a person stalking up silently behind the oblivious man. Through hazy eyes, she watched as Adelle came into focus as she drew closer. Lifting her arms high above her head, she then brought them down hard over Dalton's skull with brutal force. The crunching noise that followed after she cracked him once more made Ellora sick. Adelle's trusty bat had found its mark with practiced precision.

Dalton's body fell limply over Ellora. Gurgling noises bubbled up out of his unconscious throat. "Did I kill tha' bastard?" Adelle gritted out angrily, observing him warily before landing a swift kick to his side for good measure.

Deciding it was safe, she helped roll him off Ellora, until the exhausted girl was finally free of him. Adelle had to help her to her feet. Her adrenaline and energy reserves were completely depleted after the fight of her life. She stood on wobbly legs and immediately pulled her jeans up, thinking to herself, *I love these jeans. I'm never, ever getting rid of them,* relieved that she'd decided to put on the too-tight pants that morning.

The still-shocked girls paused long enough to look over one another, taking stock of any possible injuries. Once satisfied, Adelle wrapped her arms around her friend tightly. They let their tears take over as they cried for a brief moment. Pulling back, they thumbed away their tears, mirroring each other's actions.

Adelle tenderly kissed both Ellora's tear-stained cheeks and lifted her weapon of choice triumphantly. "I told ya once before, I'd best the Devil with this bat!" Ellora gave a weak smile, remembering their first encounter with her terrible nightmares a few months back.

Patrick and Grady raced up the stairs, bursting through the opened door. Grady could hardly breathe from the quick trek up the narrow steps. Patrick took initiative, seeing as Grady couldn't catch his breath yet. "We got a call from Gavin to check on ya, and ran up here as fast as our old legs could carry us when we were met with the sound of your shouts. Are ya a'right? Did he hurt ya at all?"

Holding Adelle's hand, Ellora nodded jerkily. "Yes, I think we're okay."

Looking down on the unconscious man lying spread eagle on the floor, Patty inquired, "This be the man you're runnin' from, Ellora?"

Nodding once, she stared down at the evil man responsible for every tragic nightmare she'd ever encountered. "Yes. This is the man responsible for it all."

Grady, finally able to speak, pointed at the frightened girls. "You two, leave us. We'll stay 'ere until the authorities arrive. Out of 'ere! Now!"

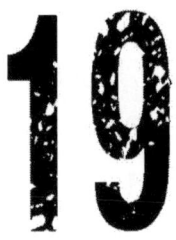

A delle and Ellora directed the authorities up the stairs while sitting huddled behind the bar, sipping some tea to warm the icy chill that the fear of the evening had brought on. They watched on at a safe distance as Dalton, who was now wide awake, was dragged out unwillingly. His eyes immediately found the green eyes he'd been searching for in the crowded room.

The wicked, eerie smile that spread across his bloodied face captured her attention, and he held her hostage with the pull of his glare. He shouted above the voices of everyone else, silencing them immediately. "I *always* win... one way or the other." His eyes stayed trained on hers as he was escorted out the door, a strange smirk plastered across his face despite his current predicament. "As long as I'm still alive, your life will belong to me. And *no one* else's."

His manic laughter echoed around the pub ominously as he kept his eyes on Ellora's until she was no longer in his sight. The sound sent icy chills down her spine. Something about his promised declaration knocked the wind out of her lungs. Something wasn't right. She fiddled with her shaky fingers as she began to pace back and forth along the length of the pub. A growing unease twisted at her insides, making her feel sick to her stomach.

Where is Behr? Hours had passed with no word. This wasn't like him at all. Surely, Gavin must've called Behr first, before calling Patrick and Grady. Something was wrong. Ellora sensed the threat deep in the marrow of her bones. Panic welled up inside her as Dalton's words replayed in her mind over and over again in a relentless, never ending loop. His threats hollowed her out, leaving behind an emptiness that had her sick with dread, fearing for the life of the only man she'd ever loved.

Had Dalton done something to hurt Behr because of her? That was something the vile snake would do to prove a point. Ellora's frame trembled as each passing moment without her love safely by her side screamed that something terrible had happened.

The pub doors opened forcefully, crashing as it swung wide, hitting the wall. Both girls jumped, startled by the sudden noise. "Behr!" Ellora cried out as tears burned behind her worried eyes, but stopped short at the sight of Gavin. Her unease escalated to panic at the absence of Behr's presence alongside his friend, after many hours had all hope draining from her weary body.

Gavin rushed toward the girls, seeing the bruising that darkened around Adelle's face, and wrapped his arms around her strongly. "My God, did he hurt you, Ellie? I'll kill 'im for layin' a hand on you!" Too emotionally exhausted to stop him, Adelle accepted Gavin's well placed kisses all along the discolored marks on her cheeks. Cupping her face delicately in his hands, he brought his mouth down to hers. His kiss unleashed all the pent up affection, frustration, and concern he'd carried around for her over the last few years, in each affectionate caress of his lips on hers.

Finally breaking the connection, Adelle answered, "No. I'm a'right. You shoulda seen the other guy."

If Ellora wasn't sure before, she definitely was now. Dalton's declaration and Behr's absence wasn't a coincidence. "Gavin? Where's Behr?"

Adelle's eyebrows lifted at the devastation in her friend's voice, and she wrapped her arms around Ellora's shoulders, trying to comfort her. Gavin dipped his head, avoiding her eyes, and that was all the confirmation she needed. Ellora's stomach plummeted, and she had to brace herself against her friend to keep from toppling over. The whole room spun wildly out of control, and she fought to keep from collapsing under the crippling weight of all the devastating scenarios Behr could've been a part of.

"Behr's Ferry was found in wreckage all along the cliff side rocks..."

Pushing past Adelle, she shouted forcefully, as hot tears streamed down her cheeks. "WHERE IS BEHR? GAVIN! WHERE IS HE?" Not wanting to accept that something happened to him, she continued to shout, pounding on his chest.

Not at all offended by her understandable outburst, Gavin wrapped his arms around her tightly, uneasiness laced with each and every word uttered. "They are looking, Lor. They won't stop looking until they find him."

Ellora's legs finally gave out on her, and she crumpled to the ground, sobbing uncontrollably. "Oh, Gavin. It's all my fault. I made him angry at me. He left because of me. Oh my God, I should've never come here. I led Dalton right to your front door." She was losing it. If anything happened to him, she would never forgive herself, and she would never recover from it.

Thoughts of having to pick up and move worked their way through her head. She wouldn't be able to remain in a place filled with such remarkable memories of the life she so desperately wanted; it would break her. But, just the idea of leaving her new family behind hurt her already torn up heart.

Ellora knew she couldn't live without Behr right beside her. She loved him so much. They had the kind of love that lasts forever... the kind of love her parents had for each other. And now, it was gone. Once again, Dalton ripped someone she loved most in the world right out of her beating heart, destroying it.

Thunderous shouts from outside the pub caught all of their attention. Ellora feared that Dalton had broken free from his captors and was coming after her. She now believed his words. So long as he was alive, he'd always come after her. She shook as the shouting edged closer to the door. Gavin stepped in front of Adelle and stood strong, ready to shield her from whatever monster came through that door.

The door burst opened and once again crashed against the wall. Both girls screamed, leaping back and away from the terrifying figure that burst through the door and charged inside.

"ELLORA!"

Blinking several times at the voice that called out her name, she sat frozen, unbelieving. She let her eyes adjust to the dark figure in the doorway.

"Oh, m'sweet Ellora." The large figure ran toward his only reason for living, who sat shivering on the cold ground, still in a state of mournful shock.

Behr. It couldn't be. This was just her mind playing cruel jokes on her. "Behr... is it really you? He... He said no one else could have me. He said he always wins... Then, when you didn't come back, I thought... I thought he took you away from me. Oh my God, Behr, are you really here?"

Behr's stomach lurched at the sight of the dazed girl rocking back and forth. Her mind was shutting down on her, unable to handle all that had happened.

He approached the trembling girl, dripping wet, completely soaked to the bone, and leaving a large puddle to collect at his feet. He took one look at the rough state of Ellora's appearance and almost died on that very spot. The men outside said Dalton had snuck into her room and attacked her. He wasn't sure what exactly happened, but the trembling, regressed, and roughed up demeanor of his petite and delicate love had him dreaming up nothing but the worst possible outcome.

Behr dropped down on his knees, crawled over to where she sat on the gritty floor, and scooped her up into his soaked arms. Not wanting to question the already violated girl in front of an audience, he carried her into the kitchen and sat her down on a stainless steel stool. Behr located the first aid kit and approached the dazed girl. Cupping her pale face with his water logged hands, Behr tilted her head up to meet his eyes.

"Did he touch you, Ellora?" The painful sorrow that shook his voice caught her attention, the agony that screamed through his pale eyes ripping her heart to shreds.

"He tried," she answered robotically, sparing him the details. Some things were better left unsaid.

"Did he hurt you?" The whole world would fall if his beloved was harmed. His strong hands carefully gripped her chin and moved her head from one side to the other, checking for any injuries.

"Some. Just a few scratches and bruises and a massive headache. Nothing an extra strength pain reliever can't handle." She forced a weak smile, trying to relieve Behr of the heavy burden of his worry.

After searching all over her face and body, he finally

pulled her into the security his arms always promised, holding her as tight as he dared, and drenching her from head to toe. "I'm so sorry, love. I should nae left you behind like I did. I shoulda been 'ere to protect you. I'll nae forgive myself. I love you. Oh, God, I love you so much." As the warmth of his body absorbed into her frozen form and thawed the numbness that kept her in a state of shock, she awoke from her nightmarish stupor. Ellora pulled back and blinked up at the owner of her heart and soul.

Realizing that it was really Behr holding her and not some apparition, or will of the mind, that he was safe, Ellora lunged at him, not caring in the least that she was now soaked. She didn't care. She never even noticed.

"When you didn't come back, I thought... I thought he killed you. Oh my God, Behr, I thought he took you from me." She climbed onto his lap and crawled into his waiting arms, needing to be closer to the man she thought she'd lost. She wrapped her arms around his thick neck, clinging to him as tightly as she was able to in her weakened condition, chanting, "I thought you were gone. I thought I'd lost you."

Behr cradled her protectively in his strong arms as she finally let the evening's events come crashing down on her. He let her get it out of her system, sobbing hysterically against his chest.

After enough time passed, Gavin and Adelle wandered back to check in on the pair. Adelle voiced softly, full of motherly concern, "How is she doing? Is she a'right?"

Behr nodded, not daring to tear his eyes off of Ellora. "She's a'right."

Gavin walked over, dropping his hand on Behr's shoulder. His eyes spoke of all the worry he'd experienced with the absence of his oldest friend. "I truly thought the worst, friend." Ellora's body quaked violently on Behr's lap as she listened to Gavin admit to the same fears she had.

Behr looked to his friend. "How did this happen, Gavin?"

"The man himself who hired the very one you fought a few months back, Dalton, has been livin' 'ere all along, watching us all and waitin' for his chance to get to Ellora. He's the owner of the warehouse she's leasin'. He used that building as a way to get closer to her. He broke into her room upstairs and waited for her return. Adelle walked in during the attack."

Adelle spoke up, proudly announcing, "Clobbered 'im good, I did, the rat bastard."

Gavin wrapped his arm around the brave girl, tucking her into his side. "The cops 'ave 'im in custody. When I spoke of my concerns for you, that's when they gave word of your wreck. That's when that Devil of a man admitted proudly in front of everyone that it was of his doing."

The soaked man held his love closer as the very real scenario of what could've happened, had Adelle not been there, played out in his mind. He should've been the one to be there. Guilt washed over him anew. He'd stormed off, leaving her to fend off the wolves herself. He swore to himself it'd never happen again. He wasn't going to be like his father was, a man who walked out just because you didn't agree or like what your girl was saying. You stay and hash it out… together.

Gavin and Adelle decided to step back out of the room, leaving them to comfort one another in privacy.

Ellora regained some of her lost composure and finally found her voice, asking, "How did it happen?"

"I'm not sure, love, but I think he sabotaged the engine and controls somehow. The Sea Witch crashed into the rocks and sank like a stone."

"He destroyed your boat? Oh my God, Behr, are you hurt?" Ellora ran her hands up and down his face, neck, chest, and back again, searching for any injuries.

"I'm a'right, love. It takes more n' a cold surf to bring me down. I'm an excellent swimmer."

"Oh, Behr, but your boat… It is your livelihood, your dream. It's destroyed now."

Behr waved his hand, stopping her from saying anymore. "I can always get another boat. Those are just things. They are replaceable. You are not. I'm sorry I shouted at you, Lor. You dinnae deserve it."

With no more tears left to fall, Ellora's voice cracked as she proclaimed to the man she came close to losing, "Behr, I love you. I'm sorry I made you angry with me. None of this would have happened had I…" Ellora never drew a breath as her fears came tumbling out of her mouth all at once.

Behr silenced her fears with each persuasive caress from his mouth to hers, pleading against her lips for her forgiveness. This despairing kiss spoke volumes of how much he needed her, how much he loved her, and how he couldn't live without her. Cupping her face, he pierced her with his persuasive gaze.

"I was nae angry with you, love. I was angry with myself. You were right all along, and I should nae o' stormed off because I dinnae like hearin' the truth. That was an ass's way out. A true man doesn't walk away. None of this is your fault. You are responsible for your actions, nae the actions of others. That man is pure evil, and you're not responsible for his evil deeds. That is on him and him alone. I will make sure he pays for every vile thing he's done."

Placing her back on solid ground, Behr pleaded his case. "Say you forgive me, my love, and I'll make peace with my parents. I'll take you to meet them. I'll take you anywhere in the world you want to go, so long as you stand by my side. I love you, Ellora Belle. I love you so much it hurts my heart to be away from you."

Ellora shook her head, placing kisses along his dampened skin and sighing his name like an answered prayer. "Oh, Behr, I need you. I don't want to be in a world without you in it. Life wouldn't be worth living... without you living it right by my side. I love you."

Behr closed his eyes at the symphony of heartfelt

words that poured out of her mouth. Behr lowered his frame down to meet his love. Running his hands through her thick black hair, he fisted it in a tight, needy grip. Tilting her head, Ellora eagerly gripped the back of her powerful man's head and guided him to her. Their lips crashed together in a whirlwind of pent up emotions, waiting to burst out. This kiss was not at all soft or tender like their usual kisses, but a mixture of desperate need, unreleased anxiety, and fearful tension. Each battled to have the upper hand as they pulled, tugged, nipped, and devoured one another in a fury.

"Oh, Behr. Don't ever leave me. It'd kill me." She sighed against his full lips.

Behr nipped on her bottom lip. "You're my beating heart. I cannae live without you, my love. You own me. Mind, body, and soul. Without you, I am just a shell o' a man." The two continued to kiss away their fears with renewed love and devotion to one another. Each one a promise of a future together.

They were forced out of their heavenly solitude by impatient law officials needing statements. Reluctantly, Behr escorted her along without breaking some kind of physical contact. Behr's hands remained laced with hers, always reassuring, always giving her the strength she needed to keep going.

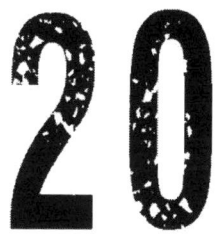

everal days had passed without a word from Dominick. After Giddeon's outburst at the prison, he probably thought he was cracking up and needed space. He didn't like the thought of letting him down, or of the detective thinking he was weak. But, for the first time in his life, Giddeon had been able to just... *be*. To breathe. To enjoy the contented bliss he'd experienced with his Angel.

They'd hardly wandered out of bed except to eat and shower. They'd spent all their time fully immersed in each other. Giddeon hadn't detected the presence of the beast within him stir, not once. The contented man let himself think that this could actually work... Him and Eva. He desperately wanted to believe that he could live a normal life, whatever that was. With her by his side, Giddeon could conquer all his demons.

As he spent the last few hours thinking of this revelation, he lay satiated with his Angel tucked close to his side. Their limbs tangled together as one, her arms draped lazily over his scarred stomach. Eva's closeness gave him a strange sense of security. He aimlessly played with her hair as she rested her head on his chest.

She hummed a soft tune as she drew imaginary figure eights over his heart. With each melody uttered, Eva drew him up out of the dark and into the light with her. The very sound of her heart thrumming along in rhythm with his chased away all the demons that had dwelled within him for so long, silencing them.

The moment Giddeon took Eva into his arms and made her his, the crack in the wall that barricaded his lifeless heart had crumbled. It was an incredible weight lifted off his shoulders. All the guilt and burdens he'd carried around for all this time had finally lifted after just one passionate encounter with his Angel. Now, he was hooked on her love, her devotion... on her.

The spent man smiled down on her as she nuzzled into his side, needing to get impossibly closer. She had spent the morning placing tender kisses on his marked up chest. Giddeon marveled at the beautiful glowing aura that radiated off of her, which was in stark contrast to his obvious darkness.

A deep sigh escaped her perfectly used lips. "I'm probably making your arm go numb." She laughed lazily as she moved to roll off him. Giddeon wrapped his arms around her as tight as he dared. Caging Eva in his demanding grasp, he rolled her onto her back. Hovering over his golden Angel, he searched over her face, marveling at all of her perfect imperfections.

With just one look, she had him drowning in the deep

blue depths of her eyes. When Eva's expressive gaze lowered to his mouth, he knew he was a goner. Without pause, Giddeon dipped his head to meet her impatient lips.

This time around, he wanted to take his time to savor the taste of her lips as they moved in exalting rhythm with his. In between kisses, Giddeon commanded, "Don't ever pull away from me, Angel. There is no better feeling in this world than the weight of your body on mine."

Pulling the woman responsible for breathing life back into him impossibly closer, Giddeon choked past his broken voice and begged against her lips, "Don't ever let me go." His words were fiercely expressed past his desperately frantic emotion, afraid that life's cruelty would take her away from him as well. His sudden anguish struck Eva like a solid blow to the chest. Her heart ached at his honest plea, triggering tears to trickle down her cheeks and onto the pillow. His worshiping caresses became more fervent, almost pleading with her not to leave him all alone in this world, like every other person that had appeared in his life had.

"I'm not going anywhere. No matter what happens," she promised determinedly, cupping his stubble roughened face in her hands. A smirk stretched across her face as she kicked the ankle monitor. "Even if you go and get lost on me, I'll still be able to find ya." She snickered when he attacked her neck, playfully nibbling the sensitive flesh like a starving dog needing a bone. Giddeon groaned as she wriggled underneath him, rousing his insatiable need for her once again.

Once again, his desire for her made its presence known. Eva stopped her movements, raising a devilish brow. "Well, looks like someone's finally waking up to join the fun," she teased.

Giddeon feasted on the delectable skin along her neck, continuing the torturous ministrations up to the earlobe that silently begged for his attention. "Mmhmm," he murmured against the soft flesh he concentrated on. The deep timber in his voice sent tremors down the length of her bare body. Chills swept through all her trembling limbs, raising goosebumps.

"I need you, Angel. Right now." Giddeon groaned as he shifted over her. Eva was anxious to feel him closer, knowing already how badly her body wanted him once more. She would never grow tired of how he made her feel.

Their bond could be described as a puzzle just shy of being complete. No other piece could ever replace the empty space. When the right pieces were finally found, they fit together so naturally, flawlessly completing the puzzle. Try with all her might to stay away… it was no use. Giddeon and Eva just fit.

In their tragically imperfect world, they made perfect sense.

Deep into their aroused haze, Eva thought she heard a faint buzzing sound. Choosing to ignore it, she wrapped her arms around his neck, pulling him closer. This time, the buzzing sounded louder, almost panicked. "Ugh!" Giddeon growled his frustration at the interruption through gritted teeth. "It's probably Dominick. He's probably freaking out. I've gotta take this."

Giddeon stretched out his arm as far as he could, unwilling to break free from Eva's embrace that kept them connected. Finally, he snatched his cell from the nightstand, reluctantly answering it. Looking down on his precious Angel, he asked harshly, "What the fuck do you want, Detective?"

A roaring engine blared offendingly in the background on the other end. "Giddeon... I've got Dalton. He was in Portree this whole time. I'm bringing him into the station now. I thought you'd like to know. It's over. We've got him. It's over." The line ended abruptly, as did all the contented peace and blissful happiness he'd cherished over the last few days.

Giddeon's short-lived carefree world was yanked out from under him at the mention of Dalton's capture. All the air was sucked out of his lungs as the now suffocating room closed in on him. Robotically, he rolled over and sat hunched over at the end of the bed.

It didn't feel over, not to him. He was supposed to be there when Dalton was captured... no one else. Giddeon had waited all this time to exact his long awaited revenge, unleash all his pent up rage, and release his wrath on the evil that had utterly destroyed his life. Instead, he'd followed his other head, straight into this girl's bed, when he was supposed to finish what he'd sought out to do from the very beginning. This wasn't right. Giddeon had to get down there before his window of opportunity was gone... forever.

Pushing himself off the bed, Giddeon stood rigidly.

Feeling the air change between them, Eva's stomach plummeted when Giddeon wouldn't even acknowledge her presence anymore. The space between them grew, as though they were miles apart, the tension in the room now thick with guilt and regret. A dreadfully nauseating sensation twisted inside her gut. "Who was that, Giddeon? What's happened?"

He continued to put the rest of his clothes on in a remarkably cold and detached way. Eva quickly snatched a t-shirt and pulled it over her head. She made her way around the bed to stand in front of the emotionally void stranger, who stood staring off at nothing. He didn't answer her, never even looked at her, as if she wasn't even in the room.

Eva's legs quaked under her as the sinking feeling of what she knew was about to happen overtook her. She marched in front of him as he tried to go. Effectively blocking his exit out, she grabbed his face in her hands, forcing him to look at her. What she observed made her sick as the acid in her stomach churned angrily inside her. Bile threatened to make its way up when she realized... *That* man was back.

Giddeon pinched his eyes closed. He couldn't look at

her when she gazed back with hurt tears glistening in her breathtaking eyes, begging for him to stay. He didn't want to hurt her, but he had to get to Dalton. He *needed* to get to Dalton. His obsessive demand for vengeance was clouding every other rational thought in his head.

A faint voice in the back of his mind spoke. "Don't go, not like this, Giddeon. Stay here with me." His growing frustration at the overwhelming need to stay against the overpowering pull to go warred inside of him. Each emotion battled to get the upper hand, leaving Giddeon's body quaking as she stood in front of him.

Trying her best to block his path, Eva shook his shoulders roughly, trying to get an answer out of the robotically numb man. Giddeon realized as he watched through a foggy haze at the stunning Angel before him, begging for some answers, he owed her that much.

Dragging his eyes off his targeted exit, Giddeon focused on her face. "They found him, Eva. The man who's responsible for butchering my parents. The man responsible for turning me into... *this*." The raw hurt that had tortured this man for countless years crashed to the surface. Giddeon threw his hands out to the side in self-disgust.

"I have to go. I promised I'd avenge them. I have to finish this." Giddeon walked forward, forcing Eva to stumble backwards as she pushed back against his solid chest. Her efforts were easily thwarted. Even her pounding fists worked to no avail, unable to halt his forward momentum.

"No, don't go, Giddeon. Don't do this. Let the detective deal with him. He's caught. They'll put him away where he'll rot, like he deserves. Don't sink to his disgusting level. It has destroyed you all these years. Can't you see that? He can't control you anymore, Giddeon, unless you let him."

Giddeon knew she would never let him leave in his current enraged state. He'd have to hurt her; that was the only way she'd let him out of the room. The thought stabbed him in the deepest part of his heart and twisted. She would never forgive him. He deserved it. He was never worthy of her anyway.

"What did you expect me to do? Move in with you? Be your fucking boyfriend? I got what I wanted from you. I'm done with you now anyway." Eva winced at the sharp edge to his biting words, like she'd been struck by them. "Your performance wasn't good enough to hold my interest, or to keep me here with you." With every vile word spewed, the short-lived warmth Eva had filled inside Giddeon's heart drained out.

Once again, his body grew cold, empty, and numb at the loss of her love that she'd poured into his heart. Eva stood frozen, her eyes wide and unblinking. New tears collected at the corners of her stunned eyes, ready to fall. Her mouth hung open at the deplorable things he'd emptied out of his mouth. After an agonizingly long and painful pause, Eva's brows dipped in righteous anger.

"I know what you're doing. Don't push me away, Giddeon. I won't back down that easily." Her voice was cracking as she forced out every word, fighting hard to keep herself from crying. Drawing in a ragged breath, she gathered up her courage and continued. "I know you feel just as strongly for me as I do for you. I know you want me just as bad as I want you." Her voice was softer when confessing her true feelings for him, and it was killing him inside.

His Angel was breaking him, and he couldn't let that happen. Pinching his eyes closed, he called upon his anger, willing it to come forward and take over. Slapping her hands away from his face, he roughly pushed past her steadfast stance.

Unwilling to give up, Eva grabbed hold of his arm and yanked back as hard as she could. "You don't need to do this! Stay with me. I know you want to stay here with me. I can feel it. I can feel your body call out to me. You need me, Giddeon. Don't be afraid to admit it. I can help get you through this."

Giddeon whirled on her, flinging the arm she held, cruelly shaking it off. "Do you help all your patients get through tough times in your bed, Counsellor? You can't save me, Eva"

His words echoed in her ears, his low blow rocking her to the core as his shouts thundered in the small room.

Standing her ground, undeterred by his growing anger, she continued. "You're right. I can't. Only *you* can do that. Fight for it, Giddeon. Fight for that second chance that's been lying in wait for you. Wake up, reach out, and take it."

The unrelenting man continued his pace down the hall with Eva following alongside, trying her hardest to get him to stop. To listen… to stay.

"It's too late for me. There's no reason for me to stay that's good enough to stop me from avenging my parents." Giddeon shook as the beast gradually took over his shell of a body. The false poison he was spewing to get her to let him go actually caused him physical pain, ripping him apart. Finally at the front door, she plastered her body against it in a last ditch effort to keep him from leaving and doing something incredibly stupid that he'd live to regret.

"Giddeon Cane… Please… Stay here. You may have lost your parents, but you still have me. I am right here. I will always stay by your side if you let me. Stay here with me." Her voice was scratchy with the hoarseness of forced back tears that burned in the back of her throat.

Her whole body trembled as she struggled to keep her composure. She wished there was a way she could shield him from all of his pain. She would take it all herself over and over again if it meant shielding him from destroying himself any farther. This man had experienced enough suffering in his life. He deserved to be relieved from it.

Giddeon clenched his fists. He'd love nothing more

than to stay right there, wrapped in her loving arms, in her warmth, and let her love drown all the demons that dwelled in the darkest parts of him. But, flashes of the look on his mother's terrified face as that man gutted her, and the hauntingly heart wrenching screams from his father as they slit her throat and dumped her lifeless body onto the floor, played out in his mind's eye.

Giddeon could still hear the weight of his father's body thump to the ground next to his beloved wife. Those unforgotten memories all but solidified his reasons for leaving. "Why would I stay here with you? I don't feel anything for you. I've gotten what you oh so willingly gave up, and I want nothing more from you. I've made my choice, *Evangelina*. And. It's. *Not.* You."

The use of her full name rendered her completely hollow inside, like someone had savagely ripped her chest open, cut out her heart, and threw it away. That raw ache is what finally broke her. With fresh tears flowing freely, she replied with a whisper, "Giddeon, your faith has been broken for a very long time, but it can still be redeemed. You can still be redeemed. You just have to want it bad enough. You have to fight harder for happiness than you have ever fought for anything else in your life. But it's worth the hardship in the end."

Giddeon's cold, unforgiving wall was brought back up, piece by piece around his heart. He reached out for the knob, easily opening the door she was trying so desperately to keep closed. Pushing past her and out the door, he destroyed the only happiness he'd ever had in his long suffering existence. "Sorry, Counsellor. I'm beyond redemption now."

The sound of her sobs quietly echoed down the building's narrow hallway. They seemed to get louder in his mind as he walked farther and farther away from her, knowing deep down he should turn around and run back to the Angel who breathed life back into his long dead heart. For a brief amount of time, he'd almost been happy. But, he knew deep down that he could never truly be happy, not until he looked upon the face of the man responsible for ripping his whole life apart and destroying it.

Eva's broken voice played out over and over in his head, the sound ringing in his ears, sealing up his heart for good. The beast, which had laid dormant for the longest period of time it ever had, was itching to claw its way back out and exact its wrath on anything within reach.

Giddeon struggled to keep himself under control. He would wait... wait until he was face to face with Dalton Ramsey Claiborne. Racing down the dew dampened sidewalk, the twisted fierce expression etched on his face gave him a sea of space as pedestrians jumped out of his way. Dalton's arrogantly smug grin flashed behind his eyes like a flickering strobe light, the image pushing his pace toward its target.

Twenty minutes later, he stormed up the stone steps

and into the main hall of the Syracuse Police Department, realizing he'd never been this desperate to get *into* a police station. After his fast paced sprint, his breathing was short and ragged, and his surreal surroundings seemed to move in slow motion.

Passing down the hall with high arched doorways, his adrenaline had spiked so high, his hearing had become fuzzy, and his sight had blurred as he struggled to regain his composure. Staggering down the hall like a drunken old man, Giddeon's heart rate elevated to an all-time high.

Somewhere inside this building, *he* was here. The obsessive need to come face to face with the man himself was unbearably overwhelming. His whole body pulsated in eagerness, ready for the attack.

Approaching a long, rich, wooden check-in desk, Giddeon's voice came out laced thick with the tension he could no longer hide. "I'm here for Detective Dominick Antonelli. Go get him and tell him Giddeon Cane is here... NOW!"

The middle-aged, red-faced man behind the desk dipped his brows in annoyance at his tone. "He's in the middle of something right now and is unavailable. What can I help you with, son?" The impatient man hopped over the desk, attracting a lot more attention from his erratic behavior as he rushed down the hall.

"HEY! You can't go back there!" Dodging a few hands that grabbed for him, Giddeon was able to avoid them all as they tried to halt him.

"Dominick! Where the fuck are you? Dominick, get out here. Don't hide him from me." A few men rushed him, grabbing him and wrenching his arms behind his back. "No! You can't do this. I just need to see Detective Antonelli. It's important. Get your fucking hands off me!"

Hearing a loud commotion, and his name being shouted over and over, Dominick leapt up out of his chair and ran to the door. He popped his head out and rushed over to the hysterical man. "It's okay, guys. He's here to see me. Sorry about this. You can let him go. I've got him." The officers pushed the unruly man toward Dominick and sauntered off.

"Giddeon, what the hell are you doing here? Have you lost your fucking mind, storming in here like that?"

The riled man approached him in a stand-off, stopping inches from his face, seething with an uncontained rage that rolled off him in waves. Through gritted teeth, he hissed out, "You *know* why I'm here. I'm not leaving until I see him. I have to confront him, and you have to let me, Detective. This may be my only chance to do it."

Dominick blew out a frustrated breath. He was stuck in between a rock and a hard place. Weighing the good and the bad of the situation, finally, he reluctantly came to a decision. He would let him see Dalton. He was, after all, locked in a holding cell until they could have him arraigned in the morning. As long as the two men stayed on opposite sides of the bars, and he had eyes on the encounter, it should be okay. If not, Dominick's ass would be on the chopping block. He was already in enough trouble as it was for making a trip out to Scotland, for the second time, without authorization.

Maybe Giddeon's presence could draw enough of a reaction out of Dalton that he would let a confession or two leak out. He'd been very tight lipped since his capture in Portree, demanding his lawyer immediately, which Dominick had expected. "Keep your fucking voice down, and try to contain yourself, and I'll let you see him. You'll have five minutes only. Try not to go fucking nuts, all right? Control yourself."

Giddeon snorted inwardly. Yeah, right. He couldn't keep that promise. "Yeah, sure. Whatever you say, Detective. Your house, your rules. Now, take me to him. I've waited long enough. My parents have waited long enough for peace."

Dominick pursed his lips tightly and nodded stiffly, motioning for the agitated man to follow him. They passed the general population holding tank, which Dalton refused to step foot in. He'd kicked up a fuss, demanding his own cell. Hoping this would get him to open up and talk more, the officers reluctantly obliged.

Giddeon could barely contain the growing rage that pulsed just below the surface. It was as though his blackened soul was moments away from bursting outward, barely contained with a desperate *need* to get to Dalton.

They finally approached a smaller cell in the very back, and Giddeon's face split into a malicious grin. Dominick crossed his arms over his chest and backed up a few steps, giving him some room. "Dalton, you have a visitor."

The marked man approached the cell like a panther stalking a caged bird. Dalton was sprawled out on the concrete slab, lounging back confidently, as though he was relaxing on his very own couch at home. Dominick gave a pointed look at Giddeon in warning. "You've got five minutes."

Dalton sat a little straighter, a broad smile stretched over his thin lips. "Aaah, the traitor has finally reared his ugly head. I have no desire to speak with the likes of this disgusting, criminal trash, Detective. I'd rather talk to an underpaid social servant, such as yourself. I have no need for this vile excuse for a human being." Looking over Giddeon, Dalton's expression was dripping with disdain. His formerly relaxed demeanor hardened the longer he stared into the malicious sneering face of his former employee.

"You really ought to have him in cuffs. I believe it is he who has committed far more violent acts than me. Just ask Ellora's parents... Oh, yeah, that's right. You can't." Dalton smiled when he was rewarded with the twisted fury in Giddeon's expression, no longer hidden. Slowly, he rose from his concrete seat, inching his way closer toward the bars. "It was you who killed them, after all… wasn't it?"

Giddeon compressed his body into the bars with bruising force, willing them to fall away and allow him access he so desperately needed inside. Reaching his arms through the bars, he situated his elbows on them, readying for a fight at a moment's notice. "Ah, yes, and I will be held accountable for my part, but you're the boss. I only did as YOU instructed me to do. Joseph and the countless others unfortunate enough to be employed by a cowardice pussy like you, or anyone else who crossed your path in a way you disliked, were all dealt with under YOUR orders."

Dalton's eye twitched at the tone and insult thrown at him. No one who valued their life dared to speak to him like that. EVER. His superior God complex commanded his movements, willing him to take a few steps closer. Dalton's transparent eyes exposed the everlasting wickedness that spread like an infectious disease deep inside his otherwise perfect outward appearance. He glared at the dirty, vile, disgraceful excuse of a man who dared to stand up to him. He wasn't even close to existing on the same level that Dalton resided.

Giddeon knew he'd hit a nerve when he glimpsed the unmistakable self-righteous wrath seething under the surface of his practiced, cool composure. Giddeon knew which buttons to push with this arrogant prick. His confident patience was slowly melting away.

Dalton clenched his shaking hands into tight fists. "I

never ordered you to mark her up, you worthless pile of human garbage. You were never to lay a hand on her. You were ordered to bring her to me... nothing more, nothing less. You're just an expendable class act, grade A, fuck up. Always have been. I thought, once upon a time, that you'd be different than all the others. You had the potential for true greatness."

Giddeon snarled, willing with all his might for Dalton to come closer to the bars. "Fuck ups, like the man who killed my parents, you mean? The men *you* hired to get everyone to vacate the property you wanted... right?"

Dalton had a brief moment of disbelief flash across his face. "How'd you find out about that... unfortunate mishap? I know it wasn't you who figured it out. You're not smart enough to solve even the smallest of problems on your own. Who told you?"

Giddeon pressed his face against the bars forcefully, wishing he could walk right through them and wrap his hands around his neck. "Everyone is rolling over on you, every single person you've kept under your controlling command. I've seen Dale. He held nothing back. I know everything."

Dalton stepped forward, not quite close enough to touch. How dare this son of a bitch question him? Dalton knew that the only way they could get Dale's name was through Susan. That disloyal, disobeying bitch would pay dearly for her traitorous backstabbing. Caught or not,

Dalton would make them all pay the price with their lives. He knew all their weaknesses. They all had them, including this pathetic looser in front of him.

"I was told that your father cried like a pathetic little girl." The suited man lunged forward, grabbing the arms that dangled through the bars and wrenching them off to the side. Now nose to nose with nothing but the bars to separate them, Dalton's voice dropped to a raspy undertone. "I was informed that he hardly put up a fight as your mother's insides spilled out all over the floor that now belongs to me. And you just hid, like the scared, pathetic little coward I know you to be. They are all dead because of your inaction. How does it feel, walking around in your cowardice, knowing that you could've done something to save them?" Dalton enjoyed toying with him, like a cat playing with his prey before devouring it.

Giddeon yanked his hands away from Dalton's grip all too easily, shaking with barely contained fury. He wrapped one hand around the back of Dalton's collared neck, forcing him to remain in place. The other gripped his throat and squeezed. Dalton sneered, showing no reaction to Giddeon's punishing stronghold, loving that he could still manipulate and control his emotions. Dalton mimicked his assailants' strike by wrapping both hands securely around the rough flesh of Giddeon's throat. Their stand-off became a game of pain tolerance. The last man standing wins.

"No. They are dead because you ordered it done.

Why'd you do it? You were rich enough to buy the land out from under all the tenants." Darkness spread over the marked up man, engulfing him in a fury that could only be quenched by spilling blood. Feeling the painful reminder of his tragic past burning a hole in his side, Giddeon released Dalton's throat and reached into his back pocket. He gripped his dagger with such brutal force, his fingernails dug harshly into his palms, anxiously readying for the right time to strike.

With a smug smile, Dalton guffawed condescendingly at his question. "Because they refused me. Who were they to refuse *me*? They were nothing. Their lives were worth even less to me." Dalton leaned forward, almost touching nose to nose, sneering in disgusted loathing. "The land was worth more to me than their meaningless lives. They were standing in the way of what I wanted. So, I had them removed... permanently."

The enraged man's strength wavered as he envisioned the twisted and horrified expressions of his parents through the eyes of a terrified boy. Seeing his moment of weakness, Dalton snarled out at him, "How's that delicious blonde counsellor of yours? Eva, is it?" Giddeon froze at the mention of her name, bringing him out of his old nightmare and thrusting him into a nightmare of a new kind. Hissing into his ear, Dalton gave him a new reason to fear him. "I will enjoy having her delicate flesh torn from her bones, and revel in the sound of her screams as I have her exterminated... nice and slow. The memory of her anguish will satisfy my amusement for years to come."

Giddeon, unable to hold himself together any longer, quaked violently as he tried so desperately to keep himself contained.

Dalton gripped his neck tighter, bringing him in closer. "I always win... one way or another. You can never beat me. I will destroy everyone around you that you care about. Not even prison can stop me. I will keep coming. I will *never* stop."

He'd heard enough and had reached his breaking point. The beast within ripped through his fragile exterior and weak control.

Pulling the dagger out of his pocket, Giddeon lunged through the bars, grabbing Dalton around the neck. His hands tightened around his throat with punishing force. Before anyone could pull him off, the bloodthirsty man brought the hand clutching the dagger up and pushed it into the flesh just above his left eye.

Dalton fought against Giddeon's hand, trying desperately to move away from the point of the blade. "Take a good look at this blade. It was the very same dagger used to murder my parents... and the very last thing you'll ever see." Giddeon pushed the blade deep into his brow and slashed viciously at Dalton's face. The unprepared man's screams echoed down the hall.

Giddeon distinguished the weight of the officers'

hands grasping him from behind, trying at no avail to pull him off the wounded prisoner. Wrapping his arm tighter around the back of Dalton's neck, he brought him in closer to his body, binding them together around the bars.

Giddeon savagely slashed at Dalton's eyes and face, digging out a deep x across the blood-stained expanse like a bullseye begging for his mark. Pressing with all his might, he watched with sick satisfaction as he split everything in its path like a hot blade through butter, reveling in the euphoric sound of Dalton's hysterical howling, as frantic hands tried fruitlessly to pull him away. With each excruciating shriek, Giddeon laughed manically, slicing the blade deeper. He wanted to make damn sure that the damage he inflicted was irreversible.

Blood oozed out of the deep wounds, marring the man's unrecognizable face. Giddeon's smile widened as he brought his face close to Dalton's ear. "Killing you wouldn't be punishment enough for all you've done. Now, your suffering will be constant. Now, you'll experience what it feels like to be imprisoned within your own body, forever blinded by darkness."

Several more officers flew in, prying Giddeon off and dragging him away from the bloodied man that lay curled up on the blood soaked concrete floor, writhing in agony. He was unaware of the countless men tackling him to the ground. Wrenching his arms behind his back, they slapped the cuffs on, but that didn't discourage the triumphant smile that snaked across his face. Closing his eyes, Giddeon enjoyed the agonizing, bellowing screams that ripped out of Dalton's lungs, and he committed each one to memory. The sound was music to his ears, and he'd be reverting back to this place in time, knowing he'd be going away for a long time for this. But it was worth it.

Finally, he'd gotten his revenge.

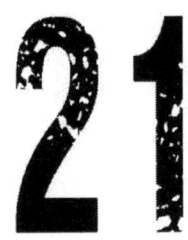

Isle of Skye,
Quairaing Mountains
Two Months Later

"We're almost there, love." Behr had picked the perfect day for their hike up the Quairaing. Clear blue skies and hardly any wind made for a perfect day to conquer the Trotternish Mountains. From ground level, the hike looked pretty intimidating, but Adelle had assured her that it was a fairly easy task. Hey, if Adelle could manage it, Ellora was sure she could, too.

It was a thirty-minute drive from Portree using the A855 Staffin Road. Surprisingly, they were able to drive a good distance up. They passed the Old Man of Storr and continued to the Quairaing gravel road-side car park. Behr pulled the truck over, and they all poured out, one by one. The gang took a moment to stretch their limbs and enjoy their surroundings.

Ellora took in the majestic beauty that surrounded her in complete awe. The rich jade green color of the impressively sized Trotternish Mountains wrapped around them on all sides. The mossy color of the steep grassy slopes climbed up the imposing rock formations that took on their unnaturally bazaar shapes. The weathered away landslide gave the ridges awe-inspiring, unbelievable silhouettes that had her imagination running wild with possible stories.

Gavin, Adelle, and Behr gathered their gear out of the back of the truck, while Ellora gazed off into the distance to where they'd be heading. Raising her hand to shield her eyes from the brilliance of the sun, she could see what looked to be an ancient looking castle. It appeared to be made of jagged volcanic rock, with high fortress walls wrapped around it, sitting atop a high cliff face.

"That is beautiful. Are we going up there?"

Behr came up behind the captivated girl, weaving his arms around her tiny waist. "Aye, that we are, love. Shouldnae take more than an hour's walk to get there." Ellora's eyes widened, shocked at the amount of time it'd take to get there. It looked to be closer than it really was.

"What is that?" She pointed at the immense nature-made structure.

Behr bent down, nuzzling into her neck, whispering low against her ear. "That there we call The Prison, and if you're a good girl an' make it up to the top, I'll have a surprise waitin' for ya."

Ellora turned into him, wrapping her arms around his neck with a challenging grin growing on her face. "Oh, is that so? Well, you've got yourself a deal."

Adelle and Gavin sidled up next to the adorable couple, handing over Ellora's pack. "We best be off. We don't want to lose the daylight." Gavin flashed Adelle a brilliant smile as he helped her with her pack, and in turn, she nodded, winking back at him. Oh, they definitely knew something Ellora didn't.

The suspicious girl snatched her pack out of his outstretched hand and began marching down the gravel path as she shouldered the heavy bag. The guys snickered at her persistence, trotting up behind her marching form.

Behr was spot on about the time it took to hike up the ridges. It took a little over an hour and a half because the girls needed to take a few short breaks to catch their breath. The elevation really sucked the oxygen out of your lungs, making even the most athletic person short winded. The trek up was steep and pretty hard to climb... but they had made it.

The views were absolutely magical. The breeze was stronger at this height, causing Ellora's midnight locks to whip around her shoulders. A faint whistling from the breeze filtered through the rocky pinnacles. "C'mon, love. Let's take a walk inside The Prison." Behr wiggled his eyebrows, with mischief dancing in his eyes. Ellora reached out and laced her fingers with his outstretched hand, following his lead.

"You can actually go inside there?"

The large man nodded at his girl. "It'll be a tight fit,

but aye, we can fit through the rock faced caverns." A wave of excited adventure rippled through her as the steep fortress walls blocked out the sun, casting dark shadows on their path. Once Behr was satisfied by how far inside he'd taken her, he halted.

Turning toward Ellora, Behr came to stand right in front of her. Without a word, he shook off his pack, dropping it to the ground. His deep blue eyes scalded hers with the heat that poured out. Cupping her delicate face with his strong hands, Behr bent down, capturing her waiting lips with his. Grasping hold of her shoulder straps, the confident man eased her heavy pack off her back and tossed it aside.

Once freed, Ellora wrapped her arms around his neck, pressing into him, needing to mold herself to his body... to bring him closer. She sighed contentedly as his hot mouth stimulated a path down the delicate flesh of her neck. Behr skimmed the roughened pads of his large hands down the delicate curve of her body, gripping her hips with mind numbing pressure. He drew her impossibly closer, into the protective warmth of his body. "I love you... so much," Behr promised in between wet kisses. "Never doubt that."

Ellora raised up on tiptoes and cupped his perfectly stubbled face. She brought him down to her and placed a soft kiss on his waiting lips, telling him without words how much she loved him back. Their mouths surged together with flawless rhythm.

Behr made sure to take his time to properly worship

her. With every stroke of the tongue or nip of her swollen bottom lip, he gave her everything. Breathless with need, he delved in deeper with the overpowering need only a man can possess, driven to consume all of her. The unmistakable desire to carry her away and finally unite their bodies into one was overwhelming. To make her his… forever.

But, the damp, narrow cavern was tight, sharp, and awkward, too awkward to take things any farther, which was exactly what they both wanted as their heated desire escalated to maddening heights.

Breaking the kiss, Behr's hands roved back up her body and cupped her face. Resting his forehead on hers, their hot breath mingled together as they panted, trying to steady their racing hearts. "C'mon, love. Let's get outta 'ere. It's time I take you to your surprise."

Ellora, dazed and lightheaded, brought her forehead against Behr's solid chest and groaned in frustration. "You mean my surprise wasn't for you to lure me into a prison and ravish me? What a bummer."

Her body moved against the vibrations of Behr's deep voice as it rumbled from laughter. "Nae, love, that was just a pleasant bonus… for me." Scooping up both their packs, Behr led the object of his affection out of the fortress walls. She reluctantly followed close behind, dragging her feet the whole way, not ready to be out of his arms so soon.

Stepping out into the bright sun from the darkness of the ancient cliff formation left her blinking rapidly in an attempt to let her eyes adjust. When the splotches faded away and her sight was back, she smiled over at her friends. Gavin definitely took full advantage of their moment alone. He had Adelle pinned against the jagged prison walls, trapping her in the cage of his arms, murmuring softly in her ear.

"What is with this place... make-out point?" Ellora muttered to herself, amused at how this spot seemed to be lust central for these Scottish boys.

Adelle was snickering as Gavin whispered something seductively into her ear. The wind whirled her strawberry locks all around them, curtaining their private moment as he tried his best to work his game on her. Adelle was a tough cookie to crack. She definitely tried her best to stay clear of his affections, but it seemed like the more she ran, the more exciting the chase was for Gavin. Ellora knew that, someday soon, Gavin would finally capture her.

Smiling at the thought, Ellora knew they'd make a fiery couple.

Grasping hold of Behr's hand, she led him away. "C'mon, let's leave them to it. They can catch up to us when they're... done." The matchmaking friend couldn't help but laugh at the last word.

Catching a sideways glimpse of his friend, Behr smiled and nodded his agreement. "Aye, love. They need some time alone."

The hiking path got really tricky after leaving The

Prison. They took the well-worn trail to the right, entering the highest point of the Quiraing. Behr led them off the beaten trail and turned left, climbing the steep earthy slope onto another narrow path. It arched its way up and to the right of the cliff side.

Ellora looked up ahead of them and spotted a narrow gap in between two towering rocky cliffs. Behr led them right through the narrow gully, climbing higher still. Once at the end, Behr hopped out of the damp gully and helped Ellora down and out of its tight path.

When she emerged from the gully, Ellora gasped in surprise at the series of well-hidden, secret paths behind the towering cliffs. "Oh, Behr, this is… this is beautiful. I have no words." The large smiling giant looked down on her with a twinkle in his eyes and an impressive smile. His masculine beauty took her breath away. The enthusiastic disposition that shown from him was a red flag to anyone who knew him. His excitement gave Behr away; they must have been close to the surprise… whatever it was.

The new path beyond the gully dropped quite dramatically. Her brute of a guide took his time climbing down, helping Ellora as she navigated her way down the slippery embankment. Behr never let her go, making sure his raven-haired beauty never stumbled. Once at the bottom, the path zigzagged around the steeper rock formations, unchanged by time. They looked as ancient as the history that surrounded them.

"This is it, love. Just over this last steep rise, and we'll 'ave arrived." Kissing her palm, Behr guided his love up the rise, slowing their pace as they neared the top. Behr climbed ahead of her, turned to face Ellora, and stopped.

Now, he was twice the height he normally was, standing on the top of the rise. As the sun shone down behind him like a historical statue, it made him look more gladiator than man, his shadow casting down on her. Behr grasped hold of both her hands, drawing her up the rest of the way. Without hesitation, Ellora stepped into him, wrapping her arms around his neck, and pressed her lips to his. She was enthralled to be up in this solitary majesty with Behr by her side.

Softly, she caressed his strong lips with hers. With no concept of time, they poured all the love, need, and lustful wanting into that kiss, melting into one another. The slide of his tongue joined with hers in a tantalizing rhythm that mimicked the kind of love they really wanted to share.

With each pass of his driving tongue, or nibble on swollen lips, the need to be as one drove them higher to a destination Ellora had yet to experience... but desperately wanted Behr to be the one to take her there. Her need to get impossibly closer to her man was stopped only by the clothes that shielded them from feeling the warmth of each other's skin.

The demand for air was the one and only thing in the world that could've separated the pair. Behr peered into the lust-hazed emerald eyes of his love. Ellora's lips curled up in a naughty tell-tale grin, breathing just as heavily as the powerful man standing over her. Their heated breath fanned over their flushed faces.

"C'mon, love." Behr pulled her up and stepped aside so she could get a look down at the impossibly enchanting view that presented itself to her. Ellora's mouth hung open in wonderment. Smack dab in the center of the tall, jagged, rocky-mountainous cliffs was an impossibly level expanse of flat, wide ground, blanketed with jade-green spongy moss.

It imitated a gigantic football field hidden in the midst of the protective Quiraing Mountains. All around it were mammoth cliff faces standing tall and proud, lining themselves all the way around the plateau. "This here... is The Table," Behr announced, sweeping his hand out and around the impressive God-made phenomenon. His deep baritone echoed around the secret location and bounced around the cliffs like a giant amphitheater.

Excitement was clearly written all over the girl's face. Ellora wanted to get down there as fast as her clumsy legs would let her. The very first thing she planned to do on the impossibly flat-leveled ground... was to call upon her inner child and execute a series off cartwheels.

Once on The Table, Ellora took a running leap and successfully executed three pinwheel cartwheels, then flung her dizzy self onto the soft spongy ground. Lying on her back, Ellora gazed up at the perfectly blue, cloudless sky. Breathing in the crisp mountain air, she let her eyes drift closed, enjoying the peaceful moment.

"Well, well, well… what is this? A lil' exercise kill your sensitive sensibilities, Yankee?" With her eyes still closed, Ellora's smile widened at the sound of Patrick's sarcastic voice as he approached.

Barely able to talk through her ceaseless snickering, Ellora answered back, "No, I could smell your stench from here and was nearly struck dead from it." Laughing along with her, Behr crouched down to pull his love up to stand.

Once up, Ellora noticed for the first time as she looked around, that her newfound family was all there—Patrick, Lachlan, Kristy, Gerard, and of course… Grady. Gavin and Adelle were finally joining the party as they climbed their way down.

Ellora nudged her best friend as she came to stand next to her. Flashing Adelle a knowing smirk, she lifted a curious eyebrow. Adelle's cheeks were flushed, lipstick gone, and her usually perfectly-in-place waves were a hot mess. When Ellora wiggled her eyebrows at her friend, all she could do was stick out her tongue.

Clearing his throat, Behr let out a rough gravelly cough. "Ellora, I have planned this out in my mind since the very moment my eyes witnessed you stumbling into Grady's Pub, and every single day since. You are always on my mind. Crawled right into the very depths of my soul, ya did. You've captured my heart and will always be its keeper. I cannae bear to be without you for even a single moment, for it truly causes me great pain." Stopping only to lace his hands through hers and kiss her knuckles, he continued. "I want you by my side through this life and the next. I love you."

Water collected in the corners of Ellora's eyes as Behr got down on one knee.

"Ellora Belle Sutherland, please do me the extraordinary honor... of being my wife." Behr reached into his pack and produced a small, black, velvet box and held it up. "In front of all our friends, family, and God's breathtaking majesty... Will you marry me?"

You could hear a pin drop as all eyes landed on Ellora. Not one person drew breath, waiting for her answer. Fresh tears of joy rolled down Ellora's shocked face. Without a word, she leapt into his arms, kissing him senseless, pulverizing his full lips, cheeks, neck, and then his waiting lips again.

Realizing, after a few of their witnesses started fake coughing, that she never actually answered his question, she shouted out, "YES! I will!"

A collective gasp and whooshing of breath that'd been held was finally unleashed at the news. The group cheered and applauded as Ellora continued to worship her very own Scottish giant with her devoted kisses.

Cupping his face, she melted into his ocean blue eyes.

"Oh, Behr, I love you so much. I couldn't imagine having any kind of future without you by my side." Lowering her voice as a rush of emotions overwhelmed her, she told him, "You're my rock, my every happiness. You have fought your way into my broken heart and made it whole. I love you."

Behr lifted his future bride and twirled her around in his arms. Kissing her through their delighted laughter, his stubble abraded her skin as he announced, "Come, Mrs. Buchanan. Let's celebrate the beginning of our forever."

Ellora followed her future husband to a large set-up of an assortment of picnic food, brought up by everyone in attendance, and ate at the most impressive table she'd ever dined on.

As the sun shone down on them all, Ellora sensed the presence of her parents right there with her. Finally, after so much time had passed, the empty hole that plagued her heart had been filled. She had an overwhelming sense that, in a way, the warmth of the sun as it wrapped itself around her was her father's way of showing that they were watching over her, and that he'd led her right to Behr.

She smiled as the voice of her father was carried along through the whistling of the mountain breeze as it circled around them, instructing Behr to take care of his little girl for him. And she knew he would. Ellora's heart was safe with him, and her life… protected.

The love that they'd found in each other was an unending love, just like the kind her parents had. And she was lucky to have stumbled into it.

EPILOGUE

Giddeon sat waiting for his first of many psych sessions he'd been court-ordered to attend. He'd gotten off a lot lighter than he anticipated after the stunt he pulled in Dalton's jail cell. He thought they would've thrown the book at him; he deserved a lot worse. Dominick really came through for him, hooking him up with a cut-throat defense attorney.

He was ordered to keep his fat mouth shut throughout the proceedings, and to just sit tight and look as pathetic and crazy as he truly was inside. He'd pleaded temporary insanity, and his experienced lawyer argued that he'd suffered through years of undiagnosed PTSD after witnessing first-hand the savage and traumatic murder of his parents. This event was a catalyst for his future that went ignored by the very state that was in charge of his well-being. He'd suffered severe depression, attempting suicide on multiple occasions, along with the abuse he'd endured from his foster parents. These events had truly shaped him into the misguided man he was today.

Yup. He was good. After all the facts were presented

against Dalton, and Giddeon's willingness to help with law enforcement, not to mention standing up to accept responsibility for his own crimes, he'd gotten off pretty light, considering. He was sentenced to two years in a super maximum security psych hospital with intense therapy, anger management, and treatment for his depression. Once released, he would be on five years' strict probation and have to continue his therapy sessions.

He was completely shocked that they didn't just lock his ass up and throw away the key, to let him rot... forgotten. The detective made good on his promise. He testified on his behalf, even though Giddeon had told him not to bother. After his sentencing, he even had it arranged to have the officer in charge of transferring him to his new home for the next two years, make a detour over to the cemetery where his parents were laid to rest.

Dominick met him there with two white roses that he handed off to Giddeon. "It's about time you visited them. Now, they can finally have peace. Let them go, Giddeon. It's over. Now's the time to better your own life. I've helped you get your second chance. Don't fuck it up." Giddeon glanced over at Dominick, who wore a smart ass grin plastered across his face. Nodding, he shook the cuffed man's hand and walked over to the parked cars to give him a moment alone.

"Detective!" Dominick whirled around to face the broken man who, in a short amount of time, had grown on him. Lifting a questioning brow, he waited.

"Thank you. For everything." The sincerity of his spoken words echoed loud and true between the two odd friends. Giddeon saluted the only man who'd ever made good on a promise and turned to face the two matching grave stones.

Kneeling at their headstones, the solemn man ran his hand down the smooth, polished stone surface. This was the first time he'd ever come to their resting place. Now, he was finally ready to accept their passing and move on from it. Bowing his head, a single tear rolled down his cheek. "I'm sorry if I've been a disappointment to you both. I remember you telling me a long time ago, Dad, that if life throws you a vicious beating, weather the storm against the ropes, and when you're presented with an opening, don't wait. Take your shot and fight back."

Giddeon placed one rose on his mother's grave, then the other on his father's. "Well, I've gotten my second chance. I won't mess it up. I'll live my life... live it for you. I love you both so much."

Giddeon quickly wiped away his stray tear when footsteps alerted him that someone approached outside the locked holding room. Following his two usual therapists was a beautiful, golden-haired Angel. She wore an infectious smile as she met his eyes. He was hit in the chest with the powerful force of his pounding heart. "Eva! What are you doing here?"

The rest of the world faded away as they regarded one another. Not an ounce of tension, anger, or awkward energy lingered between the two. The complete opposite—the air was charged with an undeniable pull that crackled like lightning around them. "I am still your counsellor, Giddeon. Detective Antonelli told your therapists that I've been of great help to you in our sessions, and he had it arranged for me to sit in on some of your sessions throughout your sentenced stay here."

Giddeon's smile widened. Dominick... that sly devil. He definitely owed him big-time. Eva was out of her usual torn jeans and t-shirt and dressed in a professional looking pencil skirt that was tight enough to leave nothing to the imagination, and a soft, delicate, silky top that accentuated every line and curve of her voluptuous figure. Her beauty left him tongue-tied. Even after everything he'd said to her, here she was, standing before him, wearing a smile that could raise the dead... and it was directed right at him. Hope crept up inside of him and grew. She was here. For him. She hadn't given up on him or walked away, like he had done to her. Her strength and unbroken promises spoke volumes to Giddeon.

But, he had to know why. Why didn't she just walk away from the train wreck that sat broken before her? "Can I talk to Eva alone for a minute? Please."

The other two looked at each other, then to Eva. She waved her hand in the air nonchalantly. "I've worked with him alone on several occasions, gentlemen. I can handle him. I only need a minute." Giddeon could tell his feisty little Angel fought to control herself from rolling her eyes at them. "I'll be all right."

They nodded at her request and gave a pointed look of warning at Giddeon. If they knew how much he treasured his Angel, they wouldn't have a reason to worry. Warily, they stepped outside. Giddeon could sense that, under the surface, they all feared him. They had been given a detailed file on him. They knew what he'd lived through, had read all the reports about the abuse he'd suffered and of all the vile things he'd done afterward. Of course, they only knew about the things he was convicted of. The rest of his demons lay hidden inside of him, where they'd stay.

Giddeon had been handled with kid gloves around this hospital, which irritated the shit out of him. No one wanted to agitate, rile, or anger him for fear of a relapse. Everyone here used quiet, expressive words and exercises to communicate. His loud cursing episodes were extremely frowned upon here.

Once the others were out of the room, Eva skipped over, grabbed a folding chair, flipped it around, and sat. Her delicate yet strong arms draped over the chair-back in front of her. "How you holding up in this nut house?" Leaning her chin on her arms, she gave him the gift of another breathtaking smile.

Giddeon sucked in a breath at the beauty of it and

sighed. He searched over her face, committing it to memory. Finally laughing at her statement, he was stunned at the music her voice made as she laughed along with him. He held nothing back, openly gazing at every line and curve of her body... remembering how she pressed against him in the blissful days he'd spent tangled up in bed with her. "Eva." Her name was a prayer that fell from his lips. "I'm... I'm sorry."

Eva interrupted him before he continued. She knew why he'd done what he did that day. No matter how misguided his intensions, she understood. Like a junkie needing a fix, he did what he had to in order to get the outcome that he needed in that moment. "Stop. You don't need to apologize to me. I know why you did it."

She paused for a moment, nibbling on her plump bottom lip, deep in thought. "The detective told me what happened. I'm glad you didn't kill him. I know that's what you sought out to do, and I know you had the opportunity."

Giddeon broke eye contact with her, running his hands through his dark, unwashed mess of hair. Ignoring her observation, he continued. "I should've never said those things... not to you." He raised his eyes, meeting hers through his thick lashes.

The brokenness and sorrow she recognized behind them stabbed at her heart.

"I'm sorry, Angel." He brought his shameful gaze back up to meet hers, their sullen surroundings falling away as they locked eyes.

"I know." Her voice cracked on the words. She wanted nothing more than to close the distance between them and wrap her arms around him. She could feel in his gaze as his eyes roamed over her that he wanted the same. But, their surroundings were heavily equipped with surveillance cameras, and their every move was being monitored.

If she wanted to keep coming back to see him like this, she'd have to watch herself. But their eyes spoke volumes, expressing everything they couldn't say out loud. "How are you doing, Giddeon... in here?" With raised eyebrows, she waited for an answer, trying desperately to change the heated atmosphere they'd created before the other two men came back in.

The corner of Giddeon's mouth turned up in a crooked smile. Tilting his head, he winked. "Best sleep I've ever had, Angel." She laughed, loving that his cocky, sarcastic nature was coming back.

"Is there anything I can get you while you're in here? Anything you need?"

Giddeon's eyes bore into hers as he slowly nodded his head. "I need to know why..." Giddeon hesitated for a moment. "Why did you agree to come out here... for me?"

Eva stood from her chair, walked over to the man who'd captured her heart, and begged to heal his. She crouched in front of him, resting her hands on his knees. "I made a promise, and I always keep my promises." Lifting a curious brow, Giddeon leaned forward, waiting for the answer.

The sound of the heavy metal door opening had them quickly standing to their feet. Before the men entered, Eva leaned in and whispered in his ear, "You told me never to pull away… and to never let you go." She brushed a feather-light kiss on his ear lobe just as the men entered, and then stepped back.

Giddeon's eyes fell closed, sealing in the memory of her whispered declaration. When he opened them, Eva was looking at him with hope for a possible future between them. With a wink, Giddeon hoped they could work on getting there while he served out his sentence. He would hold on to that hope to help him get through.

After all, it was Eva who'd declared during their session, "There is always an opportunity to change course. Your choices can take you in a completely different direction than where you were headed. You just have to have the strength to reach for it. Hold on to hope. It's as important as the air we breathe."

"All right, Mr. Claiborne, it's time to make your phone call. Make it quick." The jailor looked around, making sure the coast was clear. Dalton, with his endless means and connections, had been awarded a private phone conversation on a private line, so as not to be recorded.

"I will take all the time I need. You have no say in the matter." His hoarse voice was a threat to the guard to say no more. Once out of the infirmary, Dalton had permanently lost sight in one eye, while the other sustained lasting damage. All previous thoughts of Ellora had dissipated for the time being, in the wake of Dalton's face-off with Giddeon.

After only two rings, the line picked up. "Detective Stevens."

Dalton cleared his throat. "It's me. The time has come to call upon the favor you owe me. I need you to call my lawyer, tell him to contact Judge Rothchild immediately, and tell him all deals are off unless he gets me out. I don't care how he does it. Do it quickly and keep it quiet. I want no one to know about my release. Understood?"

Detective Stevens let out a frustrated breath. He had hoped that after hearing of his attack, he'd be free from Dalton. But nothing and no one seemed to be able to stop him. Dalton was untouchable, even in prison. The deeper Dalton pulled him into his twisted life, the farther away he was to being the upstanding peace officer he sought out to be.

"Yes, sir," was all he was able to utter.

Dalton breathed heavily into the line. "Do NOT let me down. My patience for second chances is done." The wounded man slammed the receiver down, ending the call.

Steadying his anger and regaining his composure, he struggled with his damaged sight and dialed another number. The line picked up immediately.

"I was awaiting your call. I heard what happened. What do you need me to do?" The only man Dalton could trust to get things done, Troy Wyndham, was always ready for another job.

"You have proved to be my number one after all these years. You've more than proved your loyalty to me, so you are now my right hand man. I will be entrusting you to get my affairs in order while I await my departure out of this vile place. I'm not sure how long I'll be here."

"Thank you, Mr. Claiborne." Troy's voice showed his pride in the honor bestowed to him.

Dalton knew this would please him and keep him right where he wanted him. He'd be his eyes on the outside. "I want you to place Shannon in the position Susan used to occupy as my personal secretary. Show her all that needs to be done and train her the way I like... with fear and leverage."

Dalton could almost hear him nod in satisfaction. His love of all things twisted and malicious had always appealed to Dalton's nature. "And what of the others? How would you like me to handle that... unfortunate situation?"

The blinded man engulfed in his darkness had thought on this for the last two months. "I want them all to suffer. When I get out of this disgusting place, and am set up as far away as I can get, when I give you the green light... kill them. Kill them all."

Dalton could hear the smile in Troy's voice as he agreed. "Yes, sir. It will be done. I will finish this. By the way, I have that number you asked for. It wasn't difficult to find out."

Dalton scribbled down the numbers Troy spouted off and ended the call. Dialing the last number, Dalton was delighted to hear the hesitant voice that picked up on the other end.

"Hello? Who is this?"

Dalton growled into the receiver, gripping it so tight that his knuckles whitened under the pressure.

"Game over, Susan."

To be continued in the Marked Series with
Book 3: Past Forgiven

ACKNOWLEDGMENTS

To my Lord and Savior. For he rescued us from the domain of darkness, and transferred us to the kingdom of HIS beloved Son—Colossians 1:13

To my loving Hubby. I sacrificed countless amounts of time and energy away from my family, in order to follow my dream and write this series. Your love and support means everything to me. Thank you for putting up with me. I love you so much, Eggie.

Womb-mate! Thank you so much for your continued love and support. I can always count on you. I love you, twinny.

Thanks, Mommy, for reading to us at an early age. I'm so happy I was born in a family of book lovers. Daddy, your over-exaggerated storytelling and crazy antics helped fuel my imagination.

To my Chicken Soup Chicks, thank you for always being there to help support me. You all are the best group of people on the planet. I'm truly proud and blessed to call you all my friends. I still plan on meeting you all in person someday… It'll happen.

To my Amazing Beta Readers/critique partners, Babs, Tori, and Cindi M., thank you for all your help. I'm so grateful for all your hard work. You ladies are the best! I love your faces off.

To my PA ,Tori "The Terminator" Carlson, you are a machine. Thank you for all your help, love, and support. Even with a full-time job, you're bodaciously amazeballs. You rock. The End.

Kendra, I'm so happy I've met you. Not only are you a badass editor, but I'm also happy to call you my friend.

Airicka Phoenix, once again you blew my mind with another amazing book cover and banner. I'm so in love. You did a beautiful job, and I had a blast working with you.

And last *but certainly NOT least* thank you to all my amazing readers. You are epic and I love you. Thank you for loving my characters as much as I do.

I'd love to hear from you, good or bad. Your feedback and reviews help make the next book better. THANK YOU! ~ Lady J

ABOUT THE AUTHOR

I grew up in Upstate New York, but my heart belongs in Arizona. If given the chance, I'd gladly trade in frost burn for sunburn. I grew up causing all kinds of trouble with my twin sister/partner in crime. My wild, over-exaggerated story telling grew along with my love for reading. I am a proud wife and mother of three beautiful daughters and two fur-babies.

With the support of my hubby and the encouragement of my womb-mate, I put pen to paper and let my imagination run free.

I love coffee, hiking, shooting BIG guns, and OF COURSE, reading. I enjoy all genres—paranormal, thriller, romantic suspense, dystopian... you name it.

Book One in the Marked Series, Forever Marked, released in August of 2015.

I'd love to get to know you all, so hit me up. I love to chat.

Go ahead. Don't be shy.

Where to get a hold of me:

Facebook: https://www.facebook.com/authorLadyJ

Email: LadyJauthor@yahoo.com
Goodreads: https://www.goodreads.com/LadyJ-author
Twitter: @LadyJ_Author
Instagram: @ladyj_author

KEEP READING FOR A SNEAK PEEK AT
Falling Deep Into You
(Torn Pieces: Book One)
By: Terra Kelly

Preslie was dreaming about some place warm. She was sitting on a chaise lounge reading. The back patio doors were open letting the warm air permeate the room. Then she heard an unusual sound, snoring? She looked around, but no one was there. Then the room she was in became fuzzy, and the low snoring sound became louder. She opened her eyes, adjusting them to the bright lights streaming through the windows. She was unsure at first where she was, but then her evening all came rushing back to her. She had her head still resting on Miles' leg. She looked like a cocoon, all nestled in her blanket. She knew the moment she lifted the blanket her body would feel the immediate reaction to the cool air. Unfortunately, if she waited any longer, her bladder may explode. She sighed, and carefully threw back the covers.

Trying not to startle Miles, she lifted her head slowly off his leg. She sat up, and looked over. Miles had his head to the side, and was letting out little puffs of air. Then every so often he would make a sound like a pig, and she had to quietly giggle. He was beautiful, and adorable when he slept. She let her eyes wander down to below his waistline, and sucked in air. You could see an outline, and he was very erect. So beautiful.

She sat on the edge of the couch for a few more moments, just taking in the surroundings. There was an acoustic Guitar resting against the front window, in the living room. She knew only the basics of guitars, but had always wanted to learn how to play. Looking down, she let out a soft laugh. She still couldn't believe she was wearing her most risqué nightgown. All that she had underneath was little bikini panties. She shook her head and stood up. She quietly walked to the bathroom. When she walked back into the living room, she enjoyed the feel of the soft carpet between her toes. This house was inviting. What did he say, he was renting it? It would be a keeper in her book. As she sat down on the floor, she pulled the nightgown up around her. She rested her body against the window sill, and lifted the guitar onto her lap. Her knees were together and sitting to the side in front of her. She slowly started to play a few chords.

Miles had a tough time falling asleep on the couch, but when he did, he was out. Preslie never moved the whole night, so he slept perfectly. In the past, Angie was known to toss and turn, and keep him up all night. Also, he was a light sleeper, which went with the type of job he had. You always felt on, and ready to jump into action at any moment. He never felt Preslie get up, but as he opened his eyes, he noticed she was gone. He started to come out of the sleeping fog, and realized he heard a guitar. He looked around, but didn't see Preslie. Then he looked behind him, and there she was. It was like an Angel sitting by the window. There was soft lighting shinning a beautiful beam around her gorgeous body. She was holding one of his guitars, and sitting there pretending to play. He had to smile. This was just too beautiful. The guitar she was holding was one of his prized possessions. It had been signed by Jimmy Page from Led Zeppelin. He had signed it personally. God he could watch her like this all day. He looked down and laughed to himself. Hopefully his other body parts would cooperate soon, and just relax. He couldn't stand up, when everything else was standing up, too. Shaking his head, he rubbed his eyes, and thought about cold water.

He stood and walked towards her, "Good morning, Princess."

She smiled as she looked up at him, "sorry if I woke you. I couldn't resist strumming a few chords. I really have no idea how to play, but have always wanted to learn."

Miles loved her honesty, "Well, just so happens I know this guy who plays the guitar."

Laughing, "You do, huh?" She rested her hands on the

guitar, "Was it okay that I grabbed this one?"

He sat down on the floor beside her, "Of course. Do you like Led Zeppelin?"

She looked shocked, "Who doesn't? They're the best. Why?"

He pointed down below her fingers, "Jimmy Page signed this for me. He has played on a guitar like this."

She squeaked, "Oh my God." Then she handed the guitar to him carefully, "I'm so sorry."

He let out a laugh, "Why? You didn't do anything wrong. If you were banging it around, that may be an issue." He handed the guitar back to her, and moved her hair away from her face.

He leaned in, with his head next to hers, he showed her a few notes.

She slowly moved her hands up to his, feeling each movement. She rested her head against his, and sighed.

Quietly he asked, "Should we have breakfast? Maybe wear clothes like normal people?"

He continued to strum the chords, but moved his body closer to hers. She nuzzled into the crease of his neck and rested her head on his shoulder. She lightly laughed, "Do normal people really wear clothes? In the house I mean?"

He could feel her smile on his neck, and had to smile too. "Hmmm...Maybe not." He stopped playing and moved the guitar away. He pulled her onto his lap, "Would you like to spend the day with me today?" He looked up into her eyes,

"Or do you have some reality TV show to watch?"

She playfully punched him, "No." With an innocent face, "I don't watch reality TV." You could see she wanted to laugh, but she was holding back.

He looked at her, and started laughing, "You're so lying." He shook his head, "Breakfast, then what?"

Smiling, she looked down, "Well, can we swing by my place and grab some nightgowns, or maybe clothes?" She leaned up and kissed him on his lips. Then quickly stood up, and reached for his hand.

He was a bit surprised when she leaned in to kiss him. As much as they talked in the past weeks, and especially last night. He had to get used to physical contact with another woman. After 10 years with one woman, your mind can struggle with change. Of course, Angie was making it easy to move on. He still couldn't believe he found Julian with her last night. The guys were going to freak. He looked up and grabbed her hand, and pulled himself up. He swatted her behind and walked to the kitchen.

Made in the USA
Columbia, SC
24 July 2017

Renal Diet Cookbook

*The Ultimate Easy-To-Follow Guide With
100+ Low Sodium, Low Potassium and Low
Phosphorus Healthy Recipes to Manage
Kidney Disease and Avoid Dialysis*

Table of Contents

INTRODUCTION

When it comes to your health and well-being, it's a good idea to see the doctor as often as possible to make sure you don't run into any major problems. The kidneys are your body's drug reservoir (as is the liver), cleansing the blood of foreign substances and contaminants released by food-related preservatives and other toxins.

When you eat irresponsibly and fill your body with toxins, either from food, drinks (e.g. alcohol) or even from the air you breathe (free radicals are in the sun and pass through your skin; dirty air and several foods contain them).

The body often appears to transform most substances that seem harmless until the organs of your body turn them by chemical reaction and morphing into things like formaldehyde.

For example, most of the diet sugars used in diet sodas, aspartame becomes formaldehyde in the body. These toxins must be removed or can lead to disease, kidney failure, cancer, and other painful problems.

What is kidney failure?

This is when your kidneys are unable to remove the toxins and waste in your blood from foods you eat and the things you drink. Sometimes called "chronic kidney disease" or "chronic kidney failure."

This isn't a disorder that happens overnight— it's a gradual issue that can be discovered early and treated, diet modified, and it's possible to solve what causes the problem.

Partial renal failure is possible, but it typically takes a long time (or really bad diet for a short time) to achieve full renal failure. You don't want total renal failure because it will require regular dialysis to save your life.

Specifically, dialysis procedures wash excess blood and pollutants in the blood using a device because your body can no longer do the job. Despite therapies, death could be very painful. Renal failure can result from long-term diabetes, high blood pressure, an irresponsible diet, and other health concerns.

A renal diet is about moderating the diet's protein and phosphorus intake. Limiting sodium intake is also necessary. Through regulating these two factors, you can regulate most of your body's toxins/waste which improves your kidney function.

When you notice it early enough and control your diet with extreme care, you can avoid complete renal failure. When you notice it early, you can remove it absolutely.

It's your kidney's job to remove stuff you don't need and balance the ones your body needs. If your kidneys couldn't play this role effectively, its high time you discover what you can do. A doctor's prescribed renal diet can help filter out toxic substances you don't need in your body.

A balanced kidney diet can help handle this issue.

The doctor's goal is to help remove toxic substances long before they reach your body. Through eating food, toxic substances

penetrate the skin. If you can avoid eating foods containing toxic substances, you can reduce the burden on your kidneys to flush unwanted things from your bloodstream.

A balanced renal diet implies less stress on your kidneys: apart from extracting other toxic substances like ammonia and urine, your kidneys help the body produce red blood cells and keep blood pressure stable. A doctor's prescribed diet means that your kidneys have less workload to manage.

It occurs by toxic intake monitoring. Some of the leading substances that attach toxins to your bloodstream and cause kidney problems are sodium, potassium, many proteins, and phosphorus. A doctor-monitored nutritional plan will ensure that these substances are omitted from your diet and taken in moderation.

A renal diet helps stop kidney failure progression.

You need to ensure that your kidney failure doesn't occur as a result of your kidney condition doesn't result in. A balanced healthy diet plays a major role in treating your kidney disease, so it doesn't develop out of control.

A Renal Diet helps you control phosphorous and potassium levels in your body: a healthy diet helps you limit protein to the right amount and maintain bone strength by ensuring that there is not too much phosphorus in your bloodstream. It ensures that your body system has no too much potassium because it can affect your heartbeat adversely.

A renal diet strives to ensure there is strict control of your body's sodium level to avoid water retention. If your body maintains liquids due to excessive sodium intake, you will suffer a lot of discomfort due to swelling in your leg joints. This

guide is specially written to help renal patients prepare their meals without stress; it features 100 easy and delicious renal diet recipes you can try out for your meal plan, for breakfast, lunch, dinner, and snacks.

Happy Reading!

CHAPTER 1

What is Chronic Kidney Disease?

The Function of Your Kidneys

Nephrons are the units present in each kidney which perform the basic kidney functions. We have about one million of them in each kidney.

Kidneys do a whole lot for your body, you understand. They keep our fluid accounts, balance out some of the hormones within our bodies like the parathyroid hormone, filter and clean waste, and also play a role in bone health via the processing of calcium. They also filter things like potassium.

When kidneys do not do their tasks properly, the fluid balances and processing of different wastes become considerably disturbed. This process happens over several years, or, if kidneys are injured, can quit working suddenly. That is known as acute renal failure.

Causes of Chronic Kidney Disease (CKD)

Diabetes is the number one trigger of CKD. This happens when blood glucose levels are high enough to disturb the nephrons' functions in the kidney. This is the reason the gut function is gradually reduced by diabetes that is poorly controlled.

Hypertension is another way in that the kidneys become destroyed. Since the heart's pumping action is functioning too fast in hypertension, the blood vessels are carrying repeated damage.

The blood vessels become damaged within the area of your kidneys, and wastes will be no longer be filtered. You'll have a buildup which eventually damages the kidneys.

Urinary Tract and Kidney Infections

Chronic urinary tract infections over the years will likely cause harm. Untreated Urinary Tract Diseases can travel up to the bladder area, and produce a kidney infection. Kidney infections ruin nephrons quickly, and can cause acute renal failure.

Stages of CKD

The first stage is mild harm. A blood creatinine test will demonstrate a GFR of 90-100. A GFR is also known as the glomerular filtration rate. This is a factor of how well kidneys are functioning.

It is doubtful you will notice anything at this point. Kidneys can hold up well, not working fully. Some individuals never go on to develop more stages based on their medical conditions and how well they're controlled.

In stage two of CKD, you would have a GFR of about 60-89. You likely won't have any symptoms at this stage, but occasionally protein will start showing in your pee. Urine is a good indicator of protein.

In phase three of this disease, you might observe that you are urinating often at night. It is likely you will feel fatigued, and there may be signs of anemia present. If you are experiencing cramps in the legs or itchy dry skin, then its possible that your GFR speed is under 60 at this stage.

You will need to see a nutritionist on restricting your phosphorus, potassium, and sodium, to get a diet that works. You might begin to make less urine than normal and keep fluids (edema and swelling at the extremities). Both you and your physician will begin making plans. Your GFR will likely be from 15-29, which is a large loss of kidney function.

Stage five is an advanced phase of kidney failure. Most people experience symptoms at this stage by having extreme swelling, nausea, and vomiting, and barely any urine production (possibly a teaspoonful).

Kidneys aren no longer filtering anything, and this is where you are put on dialysis for survival. Your kidney doctor will now have you keep down toxins from the bloodstream between dialysis treatments and calcium binders.

If you have hemodialysis, you will have the option of learning to do this at a center three times weekly or doing this yourself in your home. A fistula is put in the arm to get access to dialysis to wash out the blood.

Peritoneal dialysis involves the use of a catheter that is inserted into the kidney region. This is a frequent choice for most people as the constraints are not as numerous as those on hemodialysis. You do peritoneal dialysis several times daily at home, and fluids aren't as limited.

Transplants aren't always easy to comprehend, but you could always get on the list for a donor or check with family members to find out if they are donors. It is often a long process.

As you can see, the care of your kidneys is critical. It is important to have a blood test done to monitor kidney function and to work closely with your health care provider in trying to maintain kidney function.

Acute vs. Chronic Kidney Disease

The kidneys play a significant role in eliminating excessive toxins from the blood, preventing a buildup of toxic substances to levels that are harmful, and regulating calcium, sodium, and potassium levels in the blood.

A wide range of medical issues is caused when they fail to function as they need to. Determined by how it develops and the causes, kidney disease can be categorized as chronic or acute.

Acute Kidney Disease

This type develops and spreads rapidly and may go from moderate to severe within a few weeks or even days. This sometimes happens whether you have a health condition that adversely impacts the stream of urine or the supply of blood to the kidney or has an immediate impact on the organ itself. This kind is reversible. When the problem has been solved, its function goes back to normal and usually recovers completely. Sometimes, however, there might be damage that may impede functioning sometime later on.

Chronic Kidney Disease

There is a gradual loss of functioning, over time. The decline could occur over many months or even years, and the damage is usually irreversible.

The severity of this condition progresses over five quite distinct stages:

In stage one, there is moderate damage, and the organ is still working normally.

In stage two, there is a slight decrease in the efficiency with which the kidneys function.

In stage three, there is a further decrease in the operation of the kidneys. The decrease is severe and there is a near-total or complete loss of function. This is often called end-stage kidney disease. When a person reaches this point they generally need dialysis to stay alive.

Health Effects Of Kidney Disease

When the kidneys don't function as efficiently as they should, excess water, waste, and poisonous substances begin to accumulate in the bloodstream. If it is not treated in time, the kidneys will continue to deteriorate, and the toxins start accumulating to harmful levels within the body.

The buildup of toxic chemicals can cause a multitude of health problems, which range from excess or acidosis (acidity of body fluids), bone disease, anemia, and other disorders related to cholesterol and fatty acids.

Obesity is the principal element that causes kidney failure. Maintaining overall general health with a nutritious diet and exercise can go a long way.

What Are the Various Stages of Chronic Kidney Disease?

Five phases indicate kidney disorder:-

Phase one includes kidney damage with a glomerular filtration rate (GFR) at a normal or high level. There are no symptoms. Many patients won't necessarily be aware as kidneys still function.

The disease's signs include higher than ordinary levels of creatinine in blood, blood in the urine, and signs of kidney impairment in a CT scan, an MRI, or ultrasound.

Phase two includes kidney damage with a moderate decrease in their glomerular filtration rate (GFR). There may be no signs. The symptoms of phase two kidney disease include higher than ordinary levels of urea or creatinine in the blood and signs of kidney impairment in a CT or MRI scan.

Phase three includes kidney damage with a moderate reduction in the glomerular filtration rate (GFR). Because of the reduction in kidney function, most waste products accumulate in the blood. This condition is known as uremia.

Symptoms present at this phase of kidney disease include fatigue, anemia and swelling (edema) in the lower legs, kidney pain, insomnia, etc. A patient gets up at night to for urination and may urinate more or less.

The kidney now records a severe drop in the glomerular filtration rate (GFR). A patient with phase four kidney disorder

will likely require dialysis or a kidney transplant. In cases like this, a patient is likely to develop complications of chronic kidney disease like hypertension, anemia, bone disease, heart disease, etc.

Symptoms of the disease include fatigue, feeling tired, swelling (edema) of the leg; with an excessive amount of fluid, a patient could even experience breathing issues. Urine could contain blood, appearing black or fawn brown in color. Most patients do not have kidney pain, where the kidneys are present, but they might have pain in their trunk.

Phase five has the end-stage renal disease (ESRD) with a very low glomerular filtration rate (GFR). At this advanced stage, the kidneys' ability to function has dropped markedly.

Symptoms in phase five kidney disease include vomiting, nausea, swelling around the eyes and ankles, loss of appetite, headache, little or no urine, changes in skin pigmentation. The kidneys can no longer eliminate waste products from the body.

Toxins start building up in the blood that might lead to an overall feeling of malaise. Kidneys cannot perform functions like the formation of red blood cells, blood pressure regulation, and activation of vitamin D for healthy bones.

It has been observed that in many cases of chronic diabetes, too high or too low blood pressure may lead to kidney failure. Auto-immune ailments, acute infections, and uncontrolled use of chemotherapeutic medications may lead to kidneys disfunctions , which could further lead to kidney failure.

Techniques to Recognize If You are at Greater Risk of Chronic Kidney Disease

1. Having Diabetes

Diabetes is one of the most common causes of chronic kidney disease (CKD). Diabetes occurs when your body is unable to produce enough insulin or use reasonable amounts of insulin correctly.

Diabetes can cause damage to areas of the body, including the heart, kidneys, eyes, and mind. People with diabetes often develop ailments like hypertension, cardiovascular disease, chronic kidney disease, and blindness.

2. High Blood Pressure

High blood pressure or hypertension is the second top cause of CKD. This occurs when the pressure inside the blood vessels increases beyond ordinary. While this happens, the heart must work harder to pump blood through the body. Higher blood pressure may lead to chronic kidney disease, stroke, and heart attack if not controlled.

3. Family History

You may be at risk if you've got a blood relative with kidney failure. CKD runs in families; thus, if your mother, father, sister, or brother has kidney failure, you may have a greater risk.

4. Older Age (65 and over)

The elderly are a fast-growing population with a high rate of chronic kidney disease in the USA. The elderly are especially predisposed to kidney impairment because of disease and age-related decline in kidney function.

5. Ethnicity

Kidney disease is most common in Hispanic Americans, African Americans, Asian or Pacific Islanders, and American Indians. The leading cause of chronic kidney disease, diabetes, is most common in those groups.

Also, the top cause of CKD, high blood pressure, is seen in African Americans more than in any other ethnic group.

Eating Right With Chronic Kidney Disease

Particular foods should be limited if you have chronic kidney disease. There are also some foods that you could put in your diet that may help curb symptoms and avoid dialysis. If you are already on dialysis, follow the eating program provided by your physician. Before beginning any kidney disease diet, check with your healthcare professional.

It can be challenging deciding what and how to eat correctly with this disease. There are lots of foods that will need to be removed or restricted.

But, you'll also need to eat enough calories to maintain a decent energy level and stay healthy. A healthy weight has to be maintained. You do not want to lose weight since this will put you at risk for other health problems or different diseases.

Please remember to discuss your diet plans completely with your healthcare professional. Additionally, it would be advantageous to sit down and talk with a nurse or dietitian to assist with healthy choices while on the kidney disorder diet.

As a general rule, sufferers of chronic kidney disease have to restrict their intake of phosphorus and the mineral potassium. Sodium and protein will have to be consumed at carefully measured levels, and you'll want to track how much liquids you ingest.

About 5 to 7 ounces a day of high protein foods may be eaten. Protein is a tricky one as you will need enough to possess energy and fight disease, but too much can strain the kidneys. Being educated about protein foods will help in tracking them closely.

Retention can cause issues for CKD sufferers. When the kidneys are in distress, it won't be easy for them to manage an excessive amount of salt in the body—they might have to work harder to eliminate excess sodium. Limiting sodium has additional advantages like helping combat fluid retention, a problem with this disease.

Another thing to monitor closely when observing a kidney disorder diet is fluid ingestion. Talk to your doctor or dietitian; monitoring will allow you to maintain a safe quantity of fluids.

Always check with your doctor before making any changes to dieting customs or strategies. Read labels to be familiar with ingredients that are included. Eating a healthy diet can help prevent further kidney damage.

A Chronic Kidney Disease Diet Strategy For Diabetics

Out of the number of individuals who have diabetes in the United States, more than 50 percent are diagnosed with renal failure. Diabetes is the culprit. Significant changes in the blood glucose levels damage blood vessels and lower their capacity to filter the blood correctly.

The insulin imbalance also affects the nerves that signal when the bladder is full. Urinary tract ailments can be caused by the accumulation of urine in the bladder. The disease can spread to other organs if not treated. Inefficient emptying of the bladder has a negative influence on the excretory organs.

Chronic kidney disease and diabetes are a tricky combination. You require a diet program that can strike a balance between the two, one which stabilizes blood glucose levels while simultaneously ensuring a minimal buildup of waste and fluids in the body. Additionally, it also needs to be such that it fulfills your requirements.

What should you eat and what shouldn't you? I'll help you decide.

Dietary Recommendations

If you have diabetes and kidney disease, you should eat low glycemic foods. Controlling blood sugar levels helps prevent additional damage to kidneys. That is even more essential if you are currently on hemodialysis. Foods with a low glycemic index control fluid and thirst and gain and maintain a tab on blood sugar.

Fats, proteins, carbohydrates, phosphorus, potassium, and sodium should be consumed in limited amounts. It all depends on your health condition. You should reduce the intake of salty foods, legumes, and salt substitutes. Limiting salt intake decreases the amount of fluid retained by the body. Avoid adding salt to your diet when at the dining table.

Read food labels and select low-sodium options. You ought to cut back your intake of deli meats, canned foods, sauces, coatings, marinades, and toppings as they have large amounts of hidden sodium.

A good diet for kidney patients, as with a diabetic diet, focuses on protein-less foods. It is dependent on the stage of CKD, however. Individuals on dialysis can consume a more significant proportion of protein. Include poultry, fish, meats, and fat-free or skim milk.

Try as far as possible to avoid consuming diet colas, lemonades, and herbal teas since they are abundant sources of phosphorus and salt. Chronic kidney disease patients and diabetics can have a moderate amount of carbohydrates. Eat fresh fruits and vegetables rather than canned varieties.

Portion Control

Portion control is a significant aspect of a diabetic renal diet. You should control the quantity of food that you eat at every meal. A nutritionist will guide you on portion sizes that are appropriate and help you identify portion sizes.

Many times, what we believe to be one serving (restaurant size) measures as three servings. It is possible to divide the total calorie consumption into smaller meals. Eat food at regular intervals to maintain blood sugar levels.

This is a fundamental notion of food intake. If you've been diagnosed with CKD and diabetes, it is advisable to utilize a dietician to design a diet for you. Do not make any changes without first consulting a doctor, however.

Chronic Kidney Disease: What You Need to Avoid

Our kidneys are vital organs, as is our heart. Healthy kidneys are important for living well. Nowadays, there are twenty-six million Americans who suffer from CKD.

This disease can begin as early as your teens. Many folks don't even recognize they are suffering from CKD before the disease increases in intensity.

Why Do We Need Kidneys?

Kidneys are necessary because of the function they perform for our bodies, working alongside other organs within the body, acting as a filter for waste and regulating fluid. These fluids have been excreted from our urine. Equally important, our blood pressure affects our kidneys. .

What Are the Signs of Having Kidney Disease?

There are lots of trouble signs that kidney disorder is present. Bloody or discolored urine, urinary tract infections, and kidney stones are some of the indicators. All these are an early warning that, if unchecked, could be the precursor to declining health.

How Can I Test to See if I Have Kidney Disease?

There are two main tests that show if kidney disease is present. First is a urine test. Depending on protein in the urine and, more importantly, its color, your physician will have a good indication of what is happening.

Blood vessel workup may also measure kidney function. This index is called glomerular filtration speed (GFR). The filtration rate is a measure of how much flow or filtering the kidney is capable of performing, as the name implies. A GFR of less than 60mL is regarded as a powerful indicator of CKD.

Who Is At Risk of Chronic Kidney Infection?

Individuals who are already suffering from heart disease are most likely to develop CKD. Additionally, those who suffer from hypertension, obesity, or diabetes are even more prone to get to some stage of CKD.

High blood pressure puts pressure on the heart and the kidneys. Lastly, people with diabetes who don't maintain control of their glucose levels for a period will do damage to their kidneys.

How Do I Alleviate This Problem?

The reality is that other than keeping a healthy lifestyle and maintaining an appropriate weight, there is not much you can do other than to take proactive measures to protect your kidneys from the triggers of CKD. Something that will help is Omega 3 fish oil.

The fatty acids contained in ultra-refined fish oil have high levels of DHA and EPA, which have been clinically

demonstrated to help decrease inflammation. Infection is one of the damaging side effects of chronic kidney disease..

Omega 3 fish oil also acts as a natural method to deal with the disease as opposed to introducing chemicals. Dialysis is the last step short of a kidney transplant in curing this disorder.

Dialysis entails getting your blood cleansed while being hooked up to a machine. This treatment can be necessary three times a week to eradicate toxins as the liver can't perform this service.

Now that you are aware of the facts, the best defense against CKD is arresting it in the early phases by taking as much preventative action as you can. Thankfully, Omega 3 fish oil provides a natural therapy to slow down the effects of CKD.

Fish oil supplements can supply this critical line of protection. Your kidneys will remain healthier and working for years to come.

CHAPTER 2

What Is A Renal Diet?

A renal diet is an eating plan exercised to help minimize waste products' levels in the blood.

The renal diet is designed to cause as little work or stress on the kidneys as possible, while still providing energy and the high nutrients the body needs.

A renal diet follows several fundamental guidelines. The first is that it must be a balanced, healthy, and sustainable diet, rich in natural grains, vitamins, fibers, carbohydrates, omega 3 fats, and fluids. Proteins should be adequate, but not excessive.

Accumulates in the blood are kept to a minimum. Blood electrolyte levels are monitored regularly, and the diet corrected. It is essential to follow specific advice from your doctor and dietitian.

Daily protein intake is essential to rebuild tissues but needs to be kept to a minimum. Superfluous proteins need to be broken down by the body into nitrates and carbs. Nitrates are not employed by the body and have to be excreted via the kidneys.

Carbohydrates are an important source of energy and should be taken in adequate amounts. Whole grains are the best. Avoid highly refined carbohydrates.

Table salt ought to be limited to cooking only. Excess salt overworks the kidneys and causes fluid retention. Salty foods

like processed meats, lots of foods, sausages, and snacks should be avoided.

Phosphorus is essential for the body to function, but dialysis can't remove it, so amounts need to be monitored, and intake should be restricted though not eliminated completely.

Foods, like dairy products, darker drinks such as colas and legumes, have high phosphorus content. If levels of this increase in the blood, foods high in potassium such as citrus fruits and dark, leafy green lettuce, carrots or apricots might have to be restricted.

Omega 3 fats are a significant part of any healthy diet. Fish is an excellent source. Omega fats are important for the body. Avoid trans-fats or hydrolyzed fats.

Fluids should be sufficient but might need to be limited in cases of fluid retention.

A healthy renal diet can help keep kidney function for longer. The main differences between a renal diet and any nutritious diet plan are the limitations placed on protein and table salt ingestion. Restrictions on fluids and potassium might become necessary as signs and symptoms of accumulation become evident.

For people with diabetes who also suffer from kidney disease, there is a food strategy or diet. Over fifty percent of chronic kidney disease sufferers are people that have diabetes, indicating the necessity for them to stick to the diabetic diet.

In several cases, this diet is prepared and is effective in different phases of this disease. There are also instances where the diet is created for diabetics hoping to avoid renal disorder. Sufferers of

diabetes and kidney problems have trouble eating the proper food.

The aim of a diabetic's meal plan would be to get the blood within the safe selection. This may be carried out just by having meals frequently on a daily basis, not missing any, and eating carbohydrate foods that are low glycemic.

Consuming a number of such carbohydrates at every meal can assist the body in maintaining a moderate blood sugar level,becoming neither too high nor too low.

Low glycemic foods include brown rice, sweet potatoes, and whole-grain bread. But if it is a renal diet for diabetics, whole-grain bread and sweet potatoes ought not to be used since they're rich in potassium.

For people with kidney issues, they should eat less of these foods full of potassium, phosphorus and sodium. A blood sugar-lowering diet for people with diabetes can be a diet suitable for renal issues. Patients need to check labels since sodium is common in several foods.

For clients with kidney problems, dietitians advise against the consumption of diet pops of java because such drinks contain sodium.

On a diabetic-renal meal plan, unsweetened teas, water and diet sodas are allowed. When it comes to vegetables, broccoli, cauliflower, beets, eggplant, and cabbage are usually recommended because of their abundant vitamin content and very low carbohydrate and potassium content. Meats that are rich in sodium, such as organ meats, sausage, and bacon, ought not to be taken.

Since canned vegetables contain lots of sodium, it is necessary to choose raw vegetables and steer clear of the canned variety. Furthermore, raw vegetables are more nutritious, considering their vitamins.

It is recommended that diabetics learn from certified nutritionists the foods that they need to eat or avoid.

CHAPTER 3

How Renal Diets Can Make A Huge Difference In Your Day To Day Wellness

Renal diets help people with kidney disease increase their quality of life.

Other types of food may be harmful to kidneys infected with a disease, so you need to make sure you have a sound knowledge of the infection and how it affects the body.

You don't want kidney disease, but there are ways to boost your well-being by changing your diet. In reality, renal diets help you manage your health and reduce kidney disease.

You need to remember—changing your diet won't heal everybody, but it can help everyone. This doesn't mean a diet is a cure-all, so don't think of this article as medical advice; it's more of a guide.

Your doctor can provide more guidance than this does, and should always be informed or notified of any improvement in your condition.

If you have kidney problems, it's essential to regulate your health to help you feel better. There are entire books devoted to renal diets, or you can check with a registered dietitian for

recommendations. Using a Kindle or iPad, you can even download and access these books instantly.

Dietitians have experience working with those with kidney problems and can give some general do's and don'ts to follow, such as: control potassium intake—fruits like strawberries and apples are low in potassium, along with vegetables like cauliflower, cabbage and broccoli.

Track your phosphorous consumption—-creamers, pasta, cereals and rice are on the OK list.

Restrict liquid intake to 48 oz. This is the recommended level of fluid per day for renal diets—be sure to count fluid in items like grapes, ice cream, oranges, etc.

Track your salt intake—you'll need to be a tag reader to make sure you keep your salt intake low—-know what you're putting in your body and what it might contain.

Regulate your protein intake—maintain 5-7 ounces. Use egg replacements instead of normal eggs as a good technique for low protein consumption.

If you choose to use a dietitian, they can point you precisely to what you should and shouldn't consume, and why. Being aware of the effect food has on your body is important and can help you feel good every day. Also, this design is not an alternative to clinical guidelines. Yet renal diets help most kidney disease sufferers to become and stay healthier.

CHAPTER 4

An Overview of Treatment Strategies for Renal Failure

Renal failure is characterized by kidney function loss due to any number of conditions including diabetes, high blood pressure, congenital abnormalities, drug overdose, drug reactions, and many others.

Because the kidneys are the primary means of extracting excess water and waste from the bloodstream, a loss of ability can quickly lead to deadly accumulations of particles that harm vital organ systems.

Luckily, kidney failure patients have a few treatment options available that can significantly improve their quality of life and increase the number of years they have on Earth.

For those who plan to work as a technician in the dialysis industry, it is important to understand how the kidneys function and how dialysis functions, so that individuals are prepared to help answer any questions or concerns patients may have.

The kidneys are found in the lower abdominal cavity quadrant before the lower set of ribs. Such anatomical structures are about fist size and include a complex network of tubes designed to facilitate the filtration of excess water and waste from the blood, as well as absorption of inadvertently ingested nutrients.

Included in the body's vascular system is a renal artery and renal vein, responsible for directing blood to the kidneys and bringing it back to the main circulatory system.

When the heart contracts, blood passes through the complex vascular system within the kidneys and is exposed to permeable membranes containing pores wide enough to allow the passage of water and waste particles. Kidneys absorb the filtrate and transfer it to the bladder, where it is collected as urine until it can be excreted.

When the kidneys get damaged, they can no longer filter potentially harmful particles from the blood as they could when fully functional. If kidney function loss exceeds a certain percentage, individuals begin to experience uncomfortable signs and kidney failure symptoms such as water retention, nausea, and skin irritation.

At this stage, it becomes important to start exploring treatment options that can partly offset the loss in the capacity of the body to get rid of molecules it no longer needs and that could damage important organs.

The two most common treatment options are kidney transplant and dialysis therapy. Since spare kidneys can be hard to find, most patients rely on dialysis for survival while waiting for the donor's kidneys.

Dialysis is a medical procedure using a device to replicate the filtration process in a normal kidney. A dialysis patient must have a special vascular access point known as a fistula or anastomosis produced just below the skin before starting treatment. This access point links the patient to the tubes used

to transport blood from the heart to the device and back to the organ.

During each procedure, the patient sits as the device cleans the blood and adds essential nutrients that the patient may need. While the machine does a decent job of replacing a portion of the kidney filtration capacity, it cannot fully compensate for functional loss and depends on the patient's compliance with a strict renal diet for optimal health outcomes.

Some patients with renal failure are eligible for an alternative self-administered treatment called peritoneal dialysis. This blood cleaning technique uses the abdominal cavity's vascular system to remove excess water and waste. Individuals who qualify for this therapy strategy must have an abdominal wall surgically implanted pipe to attach or remove filtration fluid.

The risk factor associated with this type of dialysis is the possibility of infection of the surgical site. If this occurs, patients may have adverse side effects, and may need to go to a hospital for ongoing treatment.

CHAPTER 5

What Is Renal Dialysis?

Renal dialysis is the actual extraction technique used to selectively remove waste products and excess water from the bloodstream.

Kidneys are the filtering organs that usually perform this function. We regulate the salt, electrolyte, and fluid balance in the bloodstream necessary for all body systems to function properly.

If the kidneys become damaged or ill and their filtering ability is compromised, toxins and water accumulate in the bloodstream and poison the person if nothing is done to help them.

Renal dialysis is used as a bridging technique until either kidney functions are recovered or a kidney transplant is received.

During renal disease, the filtering system of the kidney is impaired, inefficient and inaccurate. Many molecules, such as blood cells and certain proteins, are transferred into urine and excreted, while toxic salts and water are often retained.

Renal dialysis doesn't function as well as a normal kidney, but eliminates the most toxic salts and excess water in the body.

Dialysis does not cure kidney disease, it merely conducts the essential kidney functions necessary to keep the body

functioning normally. Dialysis must be repeated at frequent intervals.

Renal dialysis, hemodialysis and peritoneal dialysis are two common types. The theory behind the dialysis is that salts and water will move through containers through a semi-permeable membrane. When the different salt solutions are combined in the right concentration, they will "catch" other salts and water.

To do this, the dialysis fluid is scientifically formulated. During hemodialysis, the patient's blood is drawn into a device via a tube during their leg. In the unit, blood flows on one side of the membrane, circulating the dialysis fluid on the opposite side and in the opposite direction. Blood is cleaned and flows back into the patient.

The process takes up to 3-5 hours and at least 2-3 times a week. Many who require hemodialysis should visit a day center where it is done. The entire procedure disrupts the dialysis patient's lifestyle.

Peritoneal dialysis usually occurs at home. This is far less disruptive for the patient, but must be done at least daily—ideally, twice daily. A special attachment is inserted into the peritoneum (abdominal cavity). The patient then removes the cap of the dialysis solution, allowing it to stream in.

The abdominal cavity's peritoneum or mucus lining is full of blood vessels, serving as the barrier between blood vessels and dialysis fluid. The liquid stays in the peritoneum for a few hours, allowing it to do its job, then is drained and disposed of. Peritoneal dialysis isn't as effective as hemodialysis, but as it's done more frequently, the results are on par.

Renal dialysis is a life-saving treatment to remove contaminants and excess fluids from the bloodstreams of patients suffering from damaged kidneys. Dialysis helps restore the electrolyte and water balance that the body needs to function properly, so patients with severe renal damage will lead relatively normal lives if their kidneys fail.

CHAPTER 6

Renal Stones

Persons with renal stones have flank pain and hematuria with or without fever. Depending on the level of the rock and the patient's underlying anatomy (for example, when only an individual working kidney is present or there is significant pre-existing renal disease), obstruction with decreased or absent urine production can make the presentation complicated.

Although a range of disorders can form renal stones, calcium is present in at least 75% of renal stones. Most calcium stones are caused by the idiopathic hypercalciuria with other major causes of hyperuricosuria and hyperparathyroidism. Uric acid stones are usually caused by hyperuricosuria, especially in persons with a history of gout, or excessive purine intake.

Deficient transport of amino acid as occurs in cystinuria may result in the creation of rock. Eventually, struvite stones composed of magnesium, ammonium and phosphate salts are a result of chronic or persistent urinary tract infections in urease-producing species.

Renal stones result from alterations in the solubility of different urine substances, such as nucleation and precipitation of salts. A number of factors can contribute to the balance of rock formation.

Dehydration encourages the formation of rocks. A high intake of fluids to maintain a normal urine volume of a few liters or

more seems protective. The exact defense mechanism is unclear.

These hypotheses include the dilution by the nephron of unknown substances predisposing to the formation of stones and the reduction of the transit time of Ca2+ that minimizes precipitation.

A high-protein diet program predisposes rock formation in sensitive individuals. A dietary protein load is responsible for intermittent metabolic acidosis and high GFR.

While Ca2 + is not detectably lower, the calcium resorption of the bone is likely transiently increased, glomerular calcium filtration is enhanced, and distal tubular calcium resorption is inhibited. For known stone formers this effect tends to be greater than in healthy controls.

A dietary plan high Na+ predisposes Ca2 + excretion and the formation of calcium oxalate, while a decreased intake of dietary Na+ has the opposite effect. In addition, urinary Na+ excretion increases monosodium urate saturation, which can be a nest for Ca2 + crystallization.

Although most stones are calcium oxalate stones, in particular, the oxalate concentration in the diet is also low to support a recommendation to avoid stone production from oxalate.

Similarly, calcium restriction, formerly the most significant dietary guideline for calcium rock formers, is only beneficial for people whose hypercalciuria relies on a diet. In other countries, decreased nutritional calcium can boost the absorption of oxalates and predispose the production of stone.

A number of elements are protective against the development of stone.

Citrate, fluids, magnesium and dietary fibers tend to have some protective effect in order to decrease in value. Forming highly soluble complexes and Chelating calcium in solution compared to calcium phosphate and calcium oxalate can prevent rock formation.

Although pharmacological dietary supplementation using potassium citrate has been shown to increase urinary citrate and pH and decrease persistent rock formation, the benefits of the naturally high-citrate dietary program have not been established. Nevertheless, some studies suggest that a lower rate of stone formation is used by vegetarians.

We probably avoid the stone-forming effects of high protein and Na+ in the diet plan, together with the protective effects of fibres. The deposition of rock in the renal pelvis is painless until a fragment breaks down and passes through the ureter, which precipitates ureteral colic. In the absence of pain, hematuria and renal damage can occur.

The inconvenience associated with renal stones is due to the ureter, renal pelvis, and renal capsule distension. The extent of the pain is related to the degree of distention that occurs and is therefore extremely highly obstructed. Anuria and azotemia suggest that a person's kidney is bilaterally obstructed or arbitrarily obstructed.

Pain, hematuria and ureteral dysfunction due to a renal stone are typically autonomous. Passage usually requires only liquids, bed rest and analgesia in smaller stones.

The principal complications are (1) hydronephrosis and permanent renal damage as result of total ureter obstruction, with resulting urine rescue and pressure build-up; (2) infection or abscess creation of a partially or entirely obstructive stone that may quickly destroy the involved kidney; (3) renal damage as a result of repeated kidney stones; and (4) hypertension.

CHAPTER 7

Acute Renal Failure - Symptoms And Treatment

Acute renal failure (ARF) is a very serious but treatable condition resulting from kidney function loss. There are various symptoms and treatments for acute renal failure or otherwise known as acute kidney failure.

What's Acute Renal Failure?

Acute kidney failure, as stated earlier, is sudden kidney function loss. As you may know, your kidneys are responsible for removing body waste products and helping balance other minerals in your body and bloodstream.

They're an essential part of the body, as the body can't work without them. In acute kidney failure, if your kidneys stop working, the body will quickly fill up with a large number of waste products, contaminants and other liquids, rendering it lethal.

How is Acute Renal Failure Caused?

Acute renal failure has various causes. Many are related to other factors in the body that can affect the kidneys, while others are directly related.

Urine-flow Blockage.

This can cause kidney failure by blocking kidney waste excretion. It can be caused by a tumour, enlarged prostate, blockage or inflammation of the urinary tract, trauma, or kidney stones.

Blood loss to the kidneys.

Any type of body injury, but more specifically localized kidney injury, can cause sudden blood flow loss, which can result in severe kidney damage. This can also be the result of a sepsis infection. Extended dehydration can cause severe damage.

Some medicines can cause acute kidney failure.

Some medicines can have some very large side effects on the kidneys. This is not a related medication, but usually from people with extended diseases. Many of these medicines can be found in some antibiotics, blood pressure medicines, certain colors used in CT scans, and more commonly some pain killers.

 All these can have a poisoning effect on the kidneys and should not be taken for extended periods. When you suffer from any of these problems, try to find other ways to cope, including finding ways to fix the first cause of the problem.

What causes acute kidney failure?

Some people may risk more acute kidney failure. For those suffering from chronic conditions such as heart conditions, obesity, liver disease, high blood pressure, and other organ conditions, they will have more chance of acute renal failure.

Also, as mentioned earlier, it is important to explore ways of reducing pressure on the kidneys when suffering from the above condition to help avoid any chances of acute renal failure or kidney disease.

What are Acute Renal Failure's common symptoms?

Before any type of kidney disease is apparent, signs can be seen and considered very mild, and some may even remain unnoticed until too late. If you have any of these common symptoms, act immediately.

Common symptoms of acute renal failure may include fluid retention (swelling in the body—usually feet and hands), loss of appetite, urinating problems, some vomiting and nausea, dizziness, lower back pain, and general restlessness.

In people already suffering from other long-term medical conditions, these signs may go unnoticed and may be thought to be related to the current disease. It is important to remember that at the slightest sign of acute renal failure symptoms, steps should be taken to help treat the condition.

Simple medical tests decide how to tell if you have acute kidney failure. After consulting the doctor, urine and blood samples must be taken.

These can help show your blood and urine toxicity and help you decide if you are now at risk of acute renal failure. Other measures, such as measuring the fluid intake and loss, are very important to help determine whether fluid retention is caused.

Acute renal failure has some forms of treatment including hospital stays and continuing procedures. All this depends on the severity of acute renal failure and signs and causes of renal problems.

Such therapies vary from dialysis, medicines, and surgery. Based on how far the renal failure can go, appropriate medication is selected.

Nevertheless, most physicians now believe that acute renal failure is largely caused by poor diet and lifestyle factors, as with virtually all medical conditions. Some of our preferred Western foods contain preservatives and chemicals that our bodies cannot process.

Along with this, they usually contain large amounts of sodium and potassium, which are not good for anyone fighting kidney disease. The kidney diet was created based on eastern diets (which now have very rare cases of genetic-related renal failure) and has been shown to help treat and even reverse acute kidney failure.

CHAPTER 8

Chronic Kidney Disease (Chronic Renal Failure/End Stage Renal Disease) And Its Dietary Management

End stage renal disease (ESRD) occurs when chronic kidney disease worsens to less than 10% of normal kidney function. The kidneys struggle to function at a day-to-day rate.

The main function of the kidneys is to eliminate waste and excess water from the body, while ESRD results in renal failure contributing to toxicity. Treatment requires kidney transplant and oral dialysis.

ESRD always follows a chronic kidney disease; the most common cause is diabetes and hypertension. Other reasons are:

1. Artery-reaching and kidney-leaving diseases

2. Congenital kidney abnormalities

3. Polycystic kidney

4. Too much pain killers or other medications

5. Toxic chemicals.

6. Autoimmune conditions including systemic lupus erythematosus (SLE)

7. Injury.

8. Glomerulonephritis.

9. Kidney stones and secondaries

10. Nephropathy reflux

11. Certain kidney disease signs include:

1. General ill-feeling, exhaustion

2. Pruritis and dry skin

3. Effortless weight loss

4. Headache

5. Appetite loss

6. Nausea

7. Diarrhea

8 Swelling

9 Bone pain

10 Bad breath

11 Abnormally dark skin. Nail changes

12. Bleeding easily—-bruises, nosebleed, stool blood

13. Impotence

14. Restless syndrome

15. Sleeplessness

16. Excessive thirst

17. Frequent hiccups

18 Amenorrhea

19. Drowsy, confused state

20. Cannot concentrate or clearly think

21. Numbness of different body parts

22. Cramps, muscle twitching.23. Decreased or no urine production.

ESRD contributes to the build-up of waste products and fluid in the body, which affects many bodily systems and functions including blood pressure regulation, red blood cell production, electrolyte balance, vitamin D and calcium levels and thus bone health.

Therefore, dialysis patients often need to undergo various tests to manage the condition:

Sodium

Potassium

Phosphorus

Calcium

Magnesium

Albumin

Cholesterol

Electrolyte

Blood count (CBC)

Erythropoietin

Parathyroid hormone

Bone density check

Care and management — ESRD management and care involves kidney transplantation and dialysis or dietary control. It is important for the patient to know and understand everything about dialysis and its forms.

Why dialysis? Dialysis helps remove and preserve the body's waste, water, and electrolyte balance. A special diet is important because dialysis alone does not effectively remove all wastes. Yet dietary control also helps minimize waste build-up and maintain water, electrolyte, and mineral balance in the body between dialysis sessions.

Patients with ESRD require high protein, low sodium, potassium and phosphorus diets and a small intake of fluids. Nevertheless, there are also drops in urine output during kidney failure.

Most dialysis patients urinate very little or not at all, so fluid restriction between treatments is very important. After urination, water builds up in the body, causing excess fluid in the chest, lungs, and ankles.

The nutritionist will measure the average amount of fluid needed based on: • Amount of urine output within 24 hours•

Level of weight gain during dialysis care • Amount of fluid retention• Dietary sodium levels • Whether you have congestive heart failure.

Tips: • Avoid or limit eating food such as soups, jell-o, popsicles, ice creams, bananas, melons, palm fruit, coconut water, cabbage, tomatoes and celery

• Smaller lenses

•Water sips

• Minimize sodium consumption

• Freeze juices in an ice tray and suck them to minimize thirst (count these ice cubes in your daily fluid intake)

• Avoid getting too hot, or going out in the sun.

Sodium balance—As above, the patient needs to avoid high sodium intake. Hypertension in ESRD is due to positive sodium balance and volume expansion (accumulation of excess fluid in the body).

 ESRD dialysis patients can effectively treat and regulate hypertension without antihypertensive drugs by having a low sodium diet (2g/day). Even a low sodium diet can make you feel less hungry, helping to stop gulping extra liquids.

Tips-• Avoid canned, processed meat.

• Avoid salt-topped foods-chips, nuts etc. • Carefully read labels;select one that reads-low sodium, no salt, sodium-free, unsalted.

• Avoid products that mention salt in the ingredient list.

- Choose food containing below 100 mg of salt per serving.

- Remove salt shaker from the table.

- Cook salt-free food instead of using flavor herbs.

- Remove dried foods—ketchup, sauces, pickles, popadums

- Do not use salt substitutes. Kidney disease also affects potassium.

Potassium balance—Usually a high potassium diet is recommended to control hypertension and thus minimize the risk of stroke and heart failure, but in the case of ESRD, a high potassium diet cannot be tolerated as these patients cannot excrete potassium from their bodies. High blood potassium levels lead to life-threatening hyperkalemia-induced arrhythmia.

Tips: • Avoid potassium-high fruits—banana, musk melons, cantaloupes, kiwis, honeydew, prunes, nectarines, coconut water, tomatoes, pineapple, lemon and orange juice, raisins and dried fruits.

- Include fruits like peaches, strawberries, pears, cherries, bananas, pineapples, plums, tangerines and watermelons.

- Avoid potassium-high vegetables—-spinach, pumpkin, squash, sweet potatoes, asparagus.

- Choose vegetables such as broccoli, cod, carrots, celery, cucumber, eggplant (aubergine/brinjal), green and waxed beans, lettuce, onion, peppers, watercress, zucchini and yellow squash.

- Avoid legumes, milk, cereal bran.

• Restrict potassium intake to 2 gm/day.

Iron — ESRD patients will also need extra iron.

Tip: • Eat a high-iron diet—lima and kidney beans, beetroot, green leafy vegetables (avoid spinach), finger millet, beef, liver, pork.

• Eat iron-fortified cereals• Take iron supplements as prescribed by your doctor.

Calcium and phosphorus—-Phosphorous levels in ESRD are elevated since our bodies cannot be excreted. Even in early renal disease, phosphorus levels may become too high.

High levels of phosphorus cause itching, vascular calcifications, secondary hyperparathyroidism, and low levels of calcium. Therefore, the calcium stored in the bones contributes to osteoporosis. A phosphate-restricted diet is recommended.

Tips: • Limit milk, yogurt, or cheese consumption.

• Can eat dairy products such as margarine, butter, cream cheese, fat cream, brie cheese and sherbet as these are low in phosphorus.

• Consult your dietician and take calcium and vitamin D supplements to help control phosphate levels.

• Avoid cane-processed food.

If phosphorus levels are not high, your doctor can prescribe phosphorus binders.

Weight control-ESRD patients lose weight without reason, so their weight must be controlled and handled with a properly

balanced diet. The average calorie intake in ESRD patients decreases to below 30-35 kcal/kg/day, leading to malnutrition.

To prevent malnutrition-related morbidity and mortality, dialysis-related ESRD patients need to undergo periodic nutrition screening and testing, comparing body weight initials with usual and ideal body weight, dietary reviews, and dietary assessment.

Protein—You must be confused when I say patients with ESRD need high protein, as a known fact is patients with renal disease should limit their protein intake. This is true as when protein breaks in our body's urea, it cannot be excreted in urine and is toxic when it builds up in the bloodstream.

A minimal protein diet is good for patient dialysis. Since protein losses in dialysis patients are higher, they need a high protein diet. In peritoneal dialysis patients, recommended dietary protein is 1.2 g/kg body weight/day and 1.2-1.3 g/kg body weight/day.

If dietary protein—calorie intake is not sufficient, patients must take dietary supplements under a nutritionist's supervision and provide tube feed or parenteral nutrition if necessary.

Tips: • Eat high-quality protein at each meal: fish, pork, eggs, kidney beans, Bengal gram, and soy.

• Add egg white or protein powder to your diet.

Carbohydrates—If you are overweight and have diabetes, you need to limit your intake of carbohydrates, but if you lose weight you need high carbohydrates. Carbohydrates are good

energy sources. The doctor or dietician will prescribe how much carbs the diet requires.

Tips: • Include fruits, vegetables, bread and grains, as they are high in fiber, minerals, vitamins and are a good energy source.

• If a high-calorie diet is advised, eat hard candy, sugar, honey, jam, pies, cakes, cookies.

• Avoid milk, chocolate, nuts and banana desserts.

Fats— ESRD dialysis patients are recommended to limit the intake of saturated fats and cholesterol as they are at high risk for coronary artery disease. We have high triglyceride levels, lower LDL (low lipoproteins) and low HDL (high lipoproteins).

Although it is recommended that you eat a high-calorie diet, you need to avoid foods that raise your triglycerides and cholesterol levels Tips:• Include foods high in monounsaturated and polyunsaturated fats and low in saturated fats. Sesame oil, flaxseeds, olive oil, and cotton seed oil.

• Avoid skin canola, coconut oil, fats, poultry and chicken.

Micronutrients—ESRDS patients are recommended for low fat diet and limited fluid intake. Thus many patients need to take a vitamin supplement as fat-soluble (A, D, E and K) vitamins and water-soluble vitamins cannot be adequately absorbed in the diet. Water-soluble vitamins are also lost during dialysis treatment. Mostly these vitamins are given intravenously through the vein during dialysis.

Managing all the above nutrients in the right quantity to suit your needs is not an easy task and cannot be achieved your own.

CHAPTER 9

Chronic Kidney Failure Diet - Is it Really Effective in Reversing Chronic Renal Failure?

Patients with chronic renal failure (CRF) are very familiar with the diet of chronic kidney failure (CKF). This diet has become so common nowadays due to increasing cases of chronic renal failure. Following this diet can help reduce the progression of your kidney disease.

CRF failure results from progressive, irreversible kidney function loss. It is typically a disease that progresses slowly over months and years depending on the kidney and the extent of the damage.

CRF has many causes, including glomerulonephritis, nephrosclerosis, obstructive kidney disorders such as kidney stones and birth defects, diabetes mellitus and systemic lupus erythematosus, and recently, illicit drugs and inappropriate analgesic use has been added.

Regardless of the cause, the outcome is the same: nitrogen waste accumulation, fluid imbalances, electrolyte deficiencies, and more. Anything is affecting multiple body systems.

It is important to stop any kidney disease progression to chronic renal failure as this would eventually lead to renal disease (ESRD). This is the phase many Americans with kidney disease fear.

The daily diet following kidney failure depends on the patient's treatment method, medical condition, and nutritional status. The following will direct your particular routine.

Dietary intervention is necessary with renal degradation and requires careful control of your protein intake, fluid intake to offset fluid losses, sodium intake to reduce sodium losses and some potassium restriction. Simultaneously, adequate caloric intake and vitamin supplementation must be ensured.

The food you consume must be of high biological quality (dairy products, eggs, meats). High biological value proteins mean complete proteins that supply the essential amino acids needed for growth and cell repair. There's plenty of kidney disease diets out there that can also help identify high biological value foods.

Generally, the liquid allowance is about 500 mL higher than 24-hour urine output the previous day. Carbohydrates and fat provide calories to avoid waste. Vitamin supplementation is essential as a protein-restricted diet does not provide vitamin supplements. Additionally, during dialysis treatment, the patient may lose water-soluble vitamins from the blood.

Chronic kidney failure diet is more than mentioned above. To emphasize it enough, it must be implemented as soon as possible to prevent further kidney damage.

CHAPTER 10

Advantages Of A Healthy Renal Diet To Kidney Disease Patient

This chapter discusses the advantages of a healthy renal diet for an individual whose kidneys are not functioning properly because of kidney disease.

Diets are made to help those suffering from a kidney disorder to live a better life.

Certain types of food may be to abnormal kidneys, so be sure to have an excellent working knowledge of not only the disease but also how it affects your body. Many people look like they are at the end of existence with their kidney disorders. This sort of diet can help you keep your kidney disease at bay and manage your well-being.

Your physician can provide you additional pointers and should always be consulted or informed of any change in your condition.

CHAPTER 11

The Ins And Outs Of A Healthy Renal Diet

When it comes to kidney health, diet goes a long way to protect your kidneys and improve their function if you are experiencing kidney damage. The best diet can vary depending upon your level of physical activity, and your level of kidney health.

While the proper diet may change depending on your kidney's condition, there are nutrients that you should know about that may need to be included or avoided on your diet and a few protocols which you could follow. Nutrition can be utilized as a form of medicine, and here we will look at dangers and the benefits of several foods.

Food And Nutrients In A Renal Diet

The subject of protein often creates a sense of confusion in regard to diet and kidney health. The best choice is to speak with your physician regarding protein requirements as they vary according to your physical activity levels, but generally speaking, if you have kidney damage, you need to limit your protein consumption.

It is suggested that dairy and red meat be excluded as sources of protein, since they are usually high in saturated fats and

sometimes sodium, which puts an extra burden upon the kidneys and cardiovascular system.

Chicken is preferable to red meat even though it is often pumped full of hormones. Fish, however, is an excellent source of protein as it is high in essential fatty acids, which are fantastic for many facets of health and have powerful anti-inflammatory properties, which can be helpful for the kidneys.

Soy proteins like tofu and tempeh are also recommended, and they have proven to help slow the progression of kidney damage if eaten regularly.

Three minerals should be avoided as part of a renal diet. That is because the kidneys need to filter these minerals from the blood, but with kidney damage this does not happen effectively, so they could build up in the blood and become dangerous.

These minerals are potassium, phosphorus, and sodium, and we will have a look at each of them.

All diets, not just the renal one, should exclude high levels of sodium. Sodium can increase blood pressure, which is not merely a danger to the kidneys but also the entire bodily system.

High blood pressure is the second top cause of kidney disease, as it forces the kidneys to filter at a higher speed, which places pressure on the kidneys over time, resulting in damage.

Additionally, kidney damage also causes high blood pressure. So we do not want to make things worse by consuming foods that increase blood pressure.

This means not adding salt to foods and avoiding takeaway and fast foods, which usually contains a lot of salt for flavoring. However, what many men and women are unaware of is that there are lots of foods that have hidden sources of sodium. These include sports drinks, canned and frozen foods, processed meats and snacks.

Potassium is another mineral that should be avoided despite being a vital nutrient required for nerve function, cardiac function, and fluid balance; however, as soon as the levels in the blood aren't adequately balanced, this presents a danger.

In the case of kidney damage, potassium levels can cause an imbalance of fluids and can build up in the bloodstream and also result in cardiovascular issues. Because of this, limiting potassium is advisable.

The extent of this will depend upon blood test results. The foods highest in potassium include: chocolate, tomato, banana, nuts, seeds, and pumpkin. In cases of too high potassium levels, it may be necessary to perform a procedure to eliminate the potassium from vegetables, since it is not feasible to avoid potassium completely.

Phosphorus should also be limited in the diet. Phosphates are found in high levels in several foods, including; dairy, wheat, milk, peanuts, legumes, chocolate, coconut, eggs, and beer.

Many of these should be avoided in a healthier diet for different reasons; it is essential to know about phosphate levels in healthy foods like eggs and legumes if magnesium levels are elevated in the blood.

Phosphorus is a vital mineral since it is involved with the regulation of calcium, and one of its primary functions is the formation of bones and teeth.

However, in the event of kidney damage, phosphorus builds up in the bloodstream and can lead to osteoporosis as it blocks absorption. Elevated levels of phosphorus can lead to high blood pressure, which, as we have found, is an extreme danger to the kidneys.

Concepts Involved In Renal Diet

One other consideration for the ideal renal diet is following an alkaline diet. Among the functions of the kidneys is balancing the pH level of the blood, which does not happen in kidney disorder. To take some of the strain off the kidneys, avoiding acidic foods is strongly recommended, and will help the kidneys to heal.

Meanwhile, acidity may contribute to a myriad of health problems throughout the body, much of which isis associated with kidney problems. The list includes kidney stones, urinary issues, high blood pressure, and poor immunity.

Now, following an alkaline diet is not as straightforward as avoiding acidic food. The residue that is left once the food is metabolized within the body, dictates whether or not that food is acidic. An example of this is lemon. It tastes acidic when digested, but it actually produces an alkalizing effect.

Generally, food items considered acidic should be avoided regardless of the diet, including carbonated snacks, beef, wheat,

alcohol, and most dairy products. However, there are foods that are a healthy component of the diet, including soy milk, fish, olive oil, and nuts.

For this diet, you need to eat 80% fatty and 20% acidic foods, which means that you may select many healthy options as part of your daily diet.

It is possible to test your urinary pH every day, and after it has shown consistent improvement, you'll be able to change into a maintenance diet of 60% alkaline and 40% acidic foods.

Alkaline foods are considered healthy as part of the renal diet plan and include fruit and vegetables, brown rice, green juices, most teas, tofu, and sprouts.

There are some specific rules which you need to know, although a diet can change depending upon the level of kidney impairment and your particular health issues.

An appropriate renal diet is vital to heal your kidneys and protect them from future harm. If you want to cure your kidneys, there are lots of herbs and nutrients that have been shown to boost kidney health.

CHAPTER 12

Formulating The Fundamentals Of A Diabetic Diet

Diabetes is the cause of renal failure; a diabetic renal diet is a critical issue. Many individuals also have diabetes. Combining a diabetic diet with a renal one has quite a few challenges. Finding an acceptable diet for kidney failure and diabetes can seem remote to the individual in the beginning.

The primary objective of a diabetic diet is to keep glucose levels at a particular level.

There are two ways of accomplishing this:

By eating carbohydrates with a low glycemic index (GI) since they're broken down and absorbed more gradually, resulting in a steady release of sugar into the bloodstream over a longer period. Low GI foods include legumes, unrefined foods, fruits and vegetables, whole grains, sweet nuts, and berries.

Highly refined and concentrated carbohydrate sugars, confectionaries, and beverages with added sugar should be avoided. They cause blood glucose "spikes" because they are very rapidly absorbed and have a tendency to burn out just as quickly.

Eating small, frequent meals (about six times a day is generally accepted). It is important to remember it is not only what is eaten, but if it is eaten, that keeps the blood glucose levels constant. Don't go long periods without eating, and don't consume huge meals or skip meals.

The diet, on the other hand, tries to limit stress on the kidneys by reducing waste products in the bloodstream:

By restricting daily protein consumption. Excess proteins have to be broken down into nitrites and carbs. The nitrites in the form of urea are eliminated in the urine. This causes unnecessary work for kidneys that are damaged.

Limiting table salt to prevent water retention. Salt replacements should not be utilized as they contain potassium.

Cutting back on other additives, such as phosphates and potassium. Frequent blood tests monitor all these and have to be restricted to the advice of your physician.

Foods with higher potassium content include banana, apricots, avocado, cantaloupe, kiwi, papaya, pears, citrus fruits, prunes, peaches, and watermelon. Some foods with high fructose content are organ meats, legumes, and dairy shellfish.

Diabetic Renal Diet:

This diet does restrict protein intake to about 8 oz, or two moderate portions, daily.

Eat only low GI carbs.

Restrict salt to cooking.

Limit foods with potassium and phosphorus content. Always follow your doctor's advice on this.

Eat small regular meals. If you wake up early in the morning, eat your first meal. Eat at 2-3 hourly intervals throughout the afternoon, taking your final meal at bedtime.

Tips:

Planning menus for a week at a time will help you change your meals.

Plan your food intake throughout the day.

When plating food for your main meal, fill the plate with vegetables or salad, then the other half with protein and carbohydrates.

Instead of salt, add flavor by using fresh herbs, onions, non-salted spices, garlic, a little lemon juice, or flavored oils.

You can enjoy whole-grain cereal, crackers or bread, fruit, a glass of skim milk, nuts, yogurt, a little cabin cheese and plenty of salads.

A diabetic renal diet can be a powerful aid in controlling both renal failure and diabetes. It is well worthwhile planning your eating and making an effort to stick to your diet. You'll feel better and be healthier because of it!

CHAPTER 13

Low Protein Renal Diet - The Best Way To Effectively Utilize It To Reverse Bipolar Disorder Progression

The low protein diet controls the intake of fluid, protein, sodium and potassium. A question often asked about this kidney diet is whether proteins are allowed. Well, the answer depends on your kidney's status.

The amount of nutrition in the diet is based on your blood levels of phosphorus, calcium, sodium, potassium, albumin, and urea. These levels are mostly measured before, during and after a dialysis treatment.

Fluid restriction relies on the quantity of weight gain and urine output between dialysis treatments. That is, whatever goes out of the body in liquid form needs to be replaced with water. Tracking your weight could be an effective practice to indicate retention that suggests kidney corrosion.

Preservation of renal function can delay the need for dialysis treatment. It can be done by controlling blood pressure and decreasing catabolism and protein intake.

A kidney patient's low protein diet depends on adjustments of components, even though there is some debate over how and

whether to keep the intake of protein of high biologic value under 50 grams, which may slow the development of renal failure.

The amount relies on how well your kidneys are working, and the quantity of protein needed to maintain health. When protein is utilized by the entire body, waste products are formed and then enter the blood.

One of these wastes is called urea. Normal healthy kidneys are good at getting rid of urea. Kidney patients should eat protein, although failing kidneys aren't good at this.

As the renal disorder progresses, the patient's ability and willingness to take in adequate nutrition diminish, and the challenge becomes to keep appropriate intake of calories but also to satisfy protein requirements.

Elemental parenteral nutrition feedings or diets may be used as well. It is essential for patients on dialysis to stick to a balance of electrolytes, minerals, and fluids.

A low protein diet should be done with the approval of your healthcare provider, who will likely be proud of you for taking a proactive approach toward your kidney disease. Bear in mind: ignorance is never an excuse for poor health habits.

Learn how to reverse your kidney disorder by following a low protein diet that has been backed by research from doctors in the nation.

CHAPTER 14

The Do's And Don'ts Of A Renal Diet

If you are currently suffering from a renal problem like kidney stones, then you should know that a renal diet plays a substantial part in preventing adverse symptoms and assisting the kidney in recuperating quickly from the issue.

While some foods could be very nutritious for your body, they may pose considerable problems to the kidneys in the long run. Because of this, patients are advised to consume foods in moderation and also evaluate the suitability of this diet to your ailment.

A renal diet should avoid calcium and phosphorous-enriched foods.

At best, dietary changes like these will become necessary if specific kidney problems are at an important stage.Below are some of the dos and don'ts that you need to think about when preparing your renal diet plan.

Don'ts of a renal diet

• Do not use food recipes in your diet that call for salts from calcium, phosphorus or manganese. These mineral components can cause kidney degeneration and handicap.

• Don't eat portions of foods that have high levels of saturated fats such as chips, hamburgers, and red meat, or any processed foods.

• Don't drink alcoholic drinks or beverages with higher sugar content—-both may overwork the liver and worsen or cause degeneration of the kidney issue.

• Don't consume sugary substances such as desserts, snacks, or candies since they cause dehydration.

• Don't take red meat on your renal diet—beef, sausage, pork, or mutton, or fried, treated, or processed meats; instead, search for lean white meat from poultry.

• Do not use any artificial sweeteners when preparing foods since they have no nutritional benefits.

• Don't use margarine or mayonnaise, but alternatives such as avocado if you want to consume fat.

• Do not eat more helpings than necessary, especially chips, ice creams, sodas, and other sweet foods, and all kinds of processed or canned foods.

• Don't eat more carbohydrates than necessary on your renal diet, including pasta, white rice or white sugar.

Do's of a renal diet

• Do take enough fluids to flush the kidney of minerals such as sodium and calcium. This will ensure proper kidney functioning, prevent dehydration, a common cause of kidney stones in the renal tubes, and detoxify the bladder.

• Do embrace a diet for the disease which contains water, whole grains, and meat and fresh vegetables. Cell metabolism and the functioning of organs improves.

• Incorporate fiber-rich foods and whole grains in your renal diet that are low in carbs but promote overall wellness and boost kidney function.

• Do create healthy eating habits to make sure that your body receives an adequate supply of minerals and nutrition.

• Do eat fruits and vegetables as often as possible and incorporate them into your renal diet plan to boost your immunity and cell metabolism.

• Do utilize low-fat milk solutions if you need to use them instead of using milk with cream or milk powder.• Fat. Lower the total amount of fat that you consume daily in your meals and when cooking.

• Do adopt an active lifestyle to combat obesity or excess weight, promote kidney functioning and proper body metabolism, and boost an effective diet. Blood circulation is improved by exercise and stimulates activities such as filtering and detoxification.

Undertaking a renal diet is important to recovery from your kidney issue. Not sticking to the instructions can cause a worsening of the problem. Seek a doctor's advice before starting any renal diet program.

CHAPTER 15

What To Eat And What To Avoid In The Renal Diet

Renal failure is defined as your kidneys not being able to put all the waste products out of your bloodstream. The waste products of course come from fluids and food the patient ingests.

I'm going to talk about what pattern or specific meal plan is suitable.

To start with is the salt intake; next is the restriction of protein, phosphorus, potassium, and fluid. Limit the intake of sodium. Yes, foods with salt are mouthwatering, but those foods do not bring you excellent benefits.

Also, the way you control your fluid intake; anything which melts at room temperature is known as fluid. Restrictions in fluid ingestion are often ordered by your healthcare provider, approximately 4 to 8 cups every day. The best way to resist thirst is to consume ice chips; that way, thirst is quenched, and the quantity of fluids is controlled.

As mentioned before, phosphorus must be restricted, particularly after dialysis is started. Dairy products, whole grains, bran, barley, nuts, coconuts, raisins, salmon, and organ meats are a few of the foods you ought to avoid.

Potassium consumption, on the other hand, has to be tapered. But what foods are high in potassium? Vegetables and fruits like pumpkin apricots, avocados, oranges, kiwi, peaches, dried fruits and nuts

Lastly, you have to consider protein restrictions in your diet regimen, even though it constitutes a portion of the patient's diet after dialysis therapy is finished. This should be undertaken with the guidance and prescription of your healthcare provider.

It is possible to have a healthy and tasty variety of meals daily, despite the restrictions. Keep these diet guidelines for renal failure in your mind, and you'll achieve several health advantages.

The kidney is a significant participant in the regulation of physiological functions. It creates a balance in the number of electrolytes in the body and also helps in filtering the blood vessels, stimulating the creation of red blood cells as well as assisting the body in getting rid of its wastes. Kidney failure occurs with the kidneys' inability to execute the functions mentioned above.

Kidney failure is a condition that is frequently a conduit for renal and urinary tract diseases. If it becomes worse, wastes can build up to high and harmful levels in your bloodstream, thereby causing complications that could include higher blood pressure, poor nutritional health, nerve damage, and anemia.

Importance Of Good Nutrition For Kidneys

A special diet is essential for individuals with kidney ailments. Eating healthy is vital to everyone but especially so for people with kidney failure. Only nutrition can give you the power to maintain a healthy weight; you need to do your activities, help build muscle, and stop infections.

Consultations with your healthcare provider can assist in advising what meals may or might not be appropriate, and a referral plan for you.

The Fundamentals Of A Great Diet For Bipolar Disorder

The basics of a healthy eating plan would be to devise a program that provides the receiver with the right quantity of vitamins, protein, minerals, and calories.

PROTEIN: Obtaining the ideal amount of protein is paramount to your general health and well-being. One of the most significant protein sources includes red meat (veal, lamb, beef), poultry, eggs, fish and other seafood, pork, grains, and vegetables.

CALORIES: Calories are the fuel our body has to produce so that we can carry out our pursuits. They allow the body to use protein up to repair the muscles and tissues in the body and help in keeping a wholesome body weight.

The quantity of calories our body needs differs from one individual to another. If you aren't getting the right number of calories into your diet, you might have to consume additional high sugary foods such as jam, syrup, honey, hard candy, etc.

MINERALS and VITAMINS: As a consequence of kidney disease and dialysis, the number of minerals and vitamins your body needs varies. As you are on a diet, you can be deprived of them by the limit on your food choices. Therefore, as recommended by your healthcare provider ONLY, you may need to take vitamins or nutritional supplements.

Controlling Other Important Nutrients

Should you suffer from kidney disease, you may want to balance electrolytes and essential minerals and fluids. These include:

PHOSPHORUS: Found in milk products, bran nuts, and drinks. An excessive amount of phosphorus in the body could result in weak bones, a build-up of calcium in the heart, blood vessels, muscles, and joints. This can ultimately lead to poor blood circulation, skin disorders, and heart conditions.

POTASSIUM: The amount of this depends on several factors that can include any drugs that may alter the levels of potassium. Excess or too little can be harmful because more potassium may be needed by some people on dialysis while less might be applicable. Excellent sources include leafy green vegetables, bananas, avocado, milk, dried beans, and legumes, etc.

CALCIUM: This is the key nutrient for building strong bones. Moreover, there is a high phosphorus content. To offset this drawback, you might need to take phosphate binders and a form of vitamin D that can be recommended by your healthcare provider.

SODIUM: This is managed by blood pressure and water balance within your body. Sodium is found in table salt, canned foods, seasoning, and meats. Lack of sodium can result in swelling of eyes, fingers, and ankles.

The kidney has a remarkable ability to recuperate from specific conditions if diagnosed early and treated with a combination of transplantation, dialysis and diet.

A diet is recommended because when problems are being experienced by your kidneys, you then start to have a decline in health. To prevent health difficulties, you need to limit your calcium intake. The majority of the kidney diet foods are a matter of substituting one food for another.

Here are some examples:

Replace dairy products with non-dairy products. Skip the milk and drink unfortified rice.

Cream cheese or cottage cheese instead of hard cheeses.

Processed grains rather than entire grains.

The best fifteen meals, which will benefit someone suffering from a kidney disorder, comprise these vegetables: rutabagas, potatoes, and winter squash rather than corn, parsnips, pumpkin seeds, or potatoes.

Vegetables include red peppers, cauliflower, cabbage, garlic, and onions. Some fruits include apples, pears, cranberries, blueberries, raspberries, strawberries, cherries, and red grapes.

Additionally, olive oil, fish, and egg whites are listed in the top fifteen.

To obtain a good kidney diet program, you need to know which foods contain less or more phosphorus. Producers have a tendency to conceal phosphorus in additives, and you must learn which take note of when you are grocery shopping.

Some examples of them are calcium phosphate, disodium phosphate, phosphoric acid, and other forms containing the phrase polyphosphates. Record the quantity of calcium so that you will learn how to recognize them; manufacturers aren't required to consider your health.

An important measure to take for yourself is to consult with a dietitian who understands your specific requirements. He will be able to help you come up with a meal program. Despite having kidney disease, your aim should still be to maintain your health. The key is to control the quantity of calcium that your body takes in.

CHAPTER 16

What Are The Advantages Of A Renal Diet?

Kidney disease is a loss of kidney function over some time, resulting in an accumulation of metabolic waste products in the body. The waste products and poisonous substances are excreted by the kidneys.

Based on the severity of this disease, kidney disease is categorized into five phases. Stage 1 is the mildest, and Stage 5 is referred to as Renal Failure. In renal failure, there is an accumulation of waste, water, and toxic substances in the body, which requires dialysis or transplantation to stay alive.

There are dietary rules to follow.

Kidneys eliminate toxins in the blood and regulate amounts of sodium, phosphorus, and potassium. In renal failure, kidneys are not able to remove metabolic waste products, and a renal failure diet helps regulate the amount of consumption of fluids, protein, sodium, potassium, and phosphorus.

PROTEIN - It is important to consume the proper quantity of protein in renal failure; the protein consumption is limited to 0.75 grams per kg body weight. Excessive consumption of protein assembles waste products in the blood, and there will

be work for your kidneys. If they're overworked in renal failure, damage to the kidneys occurs.

Less protein ingestion generates fewer waste products for the kidney, and filter function can be preserved. On the other hand, protein consumption shouldn't be too low, which can cause muscle wasting. Premium excellent sources of protein contain poultry, egg, fish, pork, and beef.

FLUIDS - It is recommended to limit fluid intake in kidney failure because excess fluid intake can lead to fluid retention. Liquid foods like soup and ice cream comprise water, and certain vegetables and fruits contain additional water, including melons, lettuce, grapes, oranges, and apples. Since they contribute to fluid retention, the consumption of foods should be monitored.

The recommended amount of fluid ingestion varies among patients. A healthcare practitioner or registered dietician can help to determine the right quantity of fluids required for a specific patient.

SODIUM - Sodium intake ought to be restricted with renal failure as it can also cause fluid retention resulting in hypertension and edema. Rich sources of sodium contain foods that are canned, processed foods, and table salt. It is advised to reduce the consumption of chips, pickles, processed cheese that was packed, meat, and junk food. Sodium intake should be less than 5 milligrams per serving.

POTASSIUM - The regular intake of potassium is 3.5 to 5.0 mEq/L, and also the intake more than the normal range should be prevented.

Kidneys excrete about 90 percent of potassium consumed through diet. Patients are recommended to restrict potassium-rich foods like milk, yogurt, citrus fruits, berries, dry fruits, bananas, beans, nuts, and legumes.

PHOSPHORUS - The ordinary ingestion of this is 2.7 to 4.6 mg/dl, and excess consumption should be avoided. Blood phosphorus levels absorb calcium from the bone and lead to bone ailments. Patients are advised to avoid phosphorous-rich foods such as cocoa, beer, dairy products, legumes, meat, and nuts.

CHAPTER 17

25 Renal Diet Breakfast Recipes

Diabetes is a medical condition whereby the body produces an inadequate amount of insulin. Insulin is a hormone. It is in charge of converting sugar, starch, and other food substance.

Renal diabetes is a sort of diabetes, which occurs because of a low-sugar threshold at the kidneys. Diabetic patients have to pay attention to their food habits. Most doctors usually prescribe a distinctive renal diet for a diabetic individual.

A renal diabetic dietary graph specifies the amount and the type of food every day that a patient should consume. A person who has renal diabetes should eat foods that contain the ideal amount of nutrients. The diets should have leguminous fruits and veggies.

Doctors also recommend a diet rich in vegetables such as cucumbers and celery, with carbohydrate amounts. Foods rich in amino acids like red beans, legumes, eggs, and lean meat are also beneficial. Food which lessens the amount of sugar in the bloodstream is beneficial in the prevention and treatment of diabetes.

It is also critical to get a diabetes patient to keep proper body weight, as it helps in controlling blood fats (cholesterol) and

lowering the blood pressure. There is a renal diet designed to make sure a person with diabetes does not gain weight.

People who have renal diabetes eat or should avoid very tiny quantities of any food that includes a high quantity of cholesterol. They should also try to lower their intake of egg yolks, fish, and fatty acids. Oil or fat used in cooking ought to be limited.

Renal diabetic patients should consume food products with reduced levels of potassium. Artichokes, Brussels sprouts, beans, lentils, lima beans, succotash, pumpkin, spinach, squash, and tomatoes are some of the vegetables present in a renal diabetic diet.

Renal diabetics can easily control their sugar level by adhering to a renal diet and leading ordinary lives.

This manual has been prepared to help renal patients prepare all foods without much hassle; it is 100+ renal diet recipes and a 30-day meal plan. Here are the foods covered in this guide:

1. 40-Second omelet

Ingredients

1 serving each recipe

Two eggs

Two tablespoons water

1 tablespoon unsalted butter

1/2 cup filling (vegetable, meat, fish)

<u>Preparation</u>

1. Beat together eggs and water until blended.

2. Inside a 10-inch omelet pan, heat the butter till it is hot enough to sizzle a water drop.

3. Pour in the egg mixture which should set at borders. Using a pancake turner, gently place the cooked portions at the edges toward the center so that the uncooked parts can reach the pan. Tilt pan and move as important.

4. Proceed until the egg is done and won't flow. If desired, fill the omelet with a half cup of vegetable, fish, poultry, or fruit filling.

5. Using the pancake turner, fold the omelet into half and invert with the bottom of the omelet.

2. 60-Second Salsa

<u>Ingredients</u>

Based on eight servings per recipe.

Four Roma or plum tomatoes, sliced

Two green onions, chopped

Three minced garlic cloves

1/2 - 1 chopped green bell pepper

1/2 - 1 new jalapeño, chopped

1/2 bunch fresh cilantro, chopped

1/2 teaspoon cumin

1/4 cup fresh oregano, chopped or one tablespoon dried

Preparation

Mix all the ingredients in a food processor or blender until the more significant items are small and chunky.

Allow it to cool for some hours inside the refrigerator.

Served chilled with tortilla chips.

3. Acorn Squash Baked with Pineapple

Ingredients

Two servings per recipe.

One acorn squash, cut in half and seeded

Two teaspoons + 1 tablespoon unsalted butter

Two teaspoons sugar

Three tablespoons pineapple

1/4 teaspoon nutmeg

Preparation

Preheat oven to 400 degrees.

Place squash in baking pan.

Place one teaspoon butter and one teaspoon sugar in each acorn half.

Cover squash with aluminum foil and bake until tender, approximately 30 minutes.

Scoop cooked squash leaving 1/4 inch shell.

Mix one tablespoon each of pineapple, pineapple butter, and nutmeg. Beat until smooth.

Spoon mixture into shells; heat at 425 degrees for about 15 minutes

4. Alaska Baked Cheese and Macaroni

Ingredients

Eight servings a recipe.

Three cups bowtie pasta shell or perhaps elbow

2 tablespoons flour

2 tablespoons butter

Two cups of milk

One teaspoon mustard powder

One teaspoon paprika

One tablespoon fresh tarragon or thyme, chopped, or perhaps one teaspoon dry

Two cups cheese (gouda, cheddar, or even other combos)

Croutons or perhaps chopped almonds

<u>Preparation</u>

Heat oven to 350 degrees.

Boil pasta until al dente in a big kettle.

Meanwhile, in a glass measuring cup, measure butter and bread. Microwave until golden brown approximately 1 or 2 minutes.

Slowly stir in milk and go on microwaving until thickened. Stir in spices and herbs.

Blend drained pasta, cheese and sauce in a greased casserole dish. Bake approximately 20 minutes.

Top with croutons and sliced almonds within the last 5 minutes.

5. Alfredo Sauce

<u>Ingredients</u>

8 servings a recipe.

1/4 cup olive oil

Three tablespoon flour

One clove garlic, minced

Two cups of rice

Four ounces cream cheese

1/3 cup shredded Parmesan cheese

1/4 teaspoon ground nutmeg

One tablespoon orange juice

Preparation

Heat organic olive oil in a skillet with average heat. Add flour and mix to create a paste. Add minced garlic.

Gradually add rice milk, whisking to avoid lumps. Let the mixture sit.

Put in cream cheese and then mix well. Remove when warm.

Include orange, nutmeg, along with 1/3 cup Parmesan cheese and juice. Blend well.

Serve with pasta, steamed vegetables, chicken, etc..

6. Almond Pecan Caramel Corn

Ingredients

Twenty cups popped popcorn or about 3/4 cup popcorn kernels

Two cups almonds

One glass pecan halves

One cup granulated sugar

One cup unsalted butter

1/2 cup corn syrup

Touch of cream of tartar

One teaspoon baking soda

Preparation

1. In a roasting pan, layer cooked popcorn with almonds and pecans.

2. Stir butter, sugar, corn syrup as well as the cream of tartar.

3. Bring the mixture to boil over medium heat, stir constantly. Let boil for five minutes without stirring.

4. Remove it from heat and stir in sodium bicarbonate.

5. Pour caramel on popcorn mixture, stirring to coat completely.

6. Bake at 200 degrees for one hour, stirring every ten minutes.

7. Let cool, stirring sometimes. Store airtight for as much as a week.

7. Anytime Energy Bars

Ingredients

8 servings a recipe.

One glass rolled oats

1/2 teaspoon ground cinnamon

3 tablespoons unsalted peanuts, chopped

1/4 glass semi-sweet mini chocolate chips

1/3 cup shredded coconut

3 huge eggs

1/3 glass applesauce

3 tablespoons of honey

Preparation

Heat oven as much as 325 degrees Celsius. Grease the pan with cooking spray.

In a mixing bowl, place chocolate chips, peanuts, cinnamon, combine yogurt, and avocado.

Beat eggs in a small mixing bowl. Insert applesauce and honey and mix well.

Add egg mixture and oats. Mix well.

Press mixture evenly in the bottom of the greased 9×9 pan.

Cook for 40 minutes. Cool, and cut into bars.

Keep refrigerated for almost 7 days.

8. Apple & Cherry Chutney

Ingredients

A moderate tart apple

One cup dried tart cherries

One little white onion, thinly chopped

One cup of apple cider vinegar

One 1/2 cup of sugar

Preparation

Cut the apple into tiny slices, leaving the apple skin on.

Set the apples and cherries in a heavy saucepan with vinegar, onion, and glucose. Mix until the sugar is dissolved and the combination begins to boil.

Cover and lower heat, cooking until the blossoms are delicate and cherries are plump and tender, for 8 10 minutes.

Set the heat very high and boil until the fruit syrup is lowered into a glaze, approximately five minutes more. Chutney may be served immediately or even maintained, covered, and refrigerated.

9. Apple and Cream Cheese Torte

Ingredients

Ten servings a recipe.

1/2 cup unsalted butter, softened

3/4 glass sugar

One glass flour

Eight ounces cream cheese

One egg

One teaspoon vanilla

3-4 moderate apples

1/2 teaspoon cinnamon

Preparation

Preheat oven to 450 degrees.

In a small bowl, cream butter as well as 1/4 cup of sugar.

Blend in flour.

Mix in a springform pan.

Beat 1/4 cup of sugar, egg, cream cheese, and vanilla until smooth.

Spread into the springform pan.

Toss apples with the remaining 1/4 cup of cinnamon and sugar.

Arrange apples on cheese filling.

Bake for ten minutes.

Reduce the oven temperature as well as bake for 25 to 30 minutes till filling is solid and apples have softened.

10. Apple Bran Muffins

<u>Ingredients</u>

Twelve servings a recipe

Two slices of whole wheat bread

One 1/2 cups wheat bran

One 1/4 teaspoon of baking soda

1/2 teaspoon nutmeg

A tablespoon of orange rind (grated)

One cup of sliced apple

1/2 glass raisins

1/2 cup of chopped nuts or perhaps sunflower seeds

Juice from one orange

Two cups of sour milk or buttermilk

A beaten egg

1/2 glass molasses

Two tablespoons of oil

<u>Preparation</u>

Preheat the oven up to 350 degrees.

Toss bran, flour, baking soda, and nutmeg, combining these with a fork.

Stir in nuts, raisins, apples, along with orange rind seeds.

Put the juice of one orange into a two-cup measure and include buttermilk to produce two cups.

Combine the buttermilk blend with oil and egg; stir completely.

Mix fluid ingredients with dry ingredients with a number of swift strokes.

Pour into greased muffin tins, then bake for twenty five minutes.

11. Apple Cup Cider

<u>Ingredients</u>

Eight servings a recipe.

2 quarts 100% apple juice

2 cinnamon sticks

1/2 teaspoon cloves, whole

One touch of nutmeg

One teaspoon allspice

Preparation

Pour apple juice and start heating.

Put in the other ingredients.

Take to a boil, then reduce heat. Let steep for ten minutes.

When prepared to serve, pour lemon using a metal sieve into a mug or thermos.

12. Apple-Filled Crêpes

Ingredients

One crêpe serving per recipe.

4 egg yolks

2 healthy eggs

1/2 glass sugar

One glass flour

1/4 glass oil

Two cups of milk

4 apples

1/2 cup unsifted sugar

1/2 teaspoon cinnamon

1/2 teaspoon nutmeg

A stick or perhaps 1/2 cup unsalted butter

Preparation

Blend egg yolks, flour, sugar, whole eggs, oil, and whole milk until batter is devoid of lumps.

Heat a little non-stick skillet over medium warmth.

Spray pan with cooking spray.

With a 2-ounce ladle spoon one or maybe 1/4 cup scoop of batter into the pan, then simply swirl the pan to distribute the crêpe batter thinly on the pan's bottom.

Cook for approximately twenty seconds. Now flip the crepe (with the help of a rubber spatula) as well as cook for approximately 10 seconds. Set crêpes separate while doing the filling.

Peel, core, as well as slice apples into twelve slices each.

Heat a medium sauté pan.

Melt butter, then add brown sugar.

Toss in the apples, nutmeg, and cinnamon.

Cook apples until tender but not soft. Set aside to cool.

To assemble the crêpes: complete the middle of each crêpe around with approximately two tablespoons of apple filling.

Roll right into a log.

13. Apple Rice Salad

<u>Ingredients</u>

Four servings a recipe.

Two cups cooked rice (any kind), chilled

Two cups (approximately 2 medium) apples, chopped

1/2 glass celery, thinly sliced

Two tablespoons unsalted sunflower seeds, shelled

2 tablespoons balsamic vinegar

One tablespoon olive oil

Two teaspoons honey

2 teaspoons dijon mustard or perhaps brown

Two teaspoons orange peel, finely shredded

One teaspoon garlic, minced

<u>Preparation</u>

Incorporate chilled rice, celery, apple, along with sunflower seeds in a big bowl.

In a small bowl, add all the remaining ingredients.

Put over the rice mixture and toss to coat.Cover and refrigerate for as much as twenty four hours before serving.

14. Asiatic Pear Crisp

Ingredients

6-8 servings a recipe.

3/4 glass nuts

1/2 cup unbleached all purpose flour

1/4 cup light brown sugar

Four tablespoons granulated sugar, divided

1/4 teaspoon ground cinnamon

1/8 teaspoon ground nutmeg

5 tablespoons unsalted butter

One tablespoon cornstarch

Liquid from a single lemon

Three lbs. Asian pears, cored and peeled

Preparation

Preheat oven to 375 degrees.

Mix nuts, flour, brown sugar, granulated sugar, cinnamon, and nutmeg for a food processor.

Pour melted butter until the mixture looks like damp sand.

Whisk remaining two tablespoons granulated sugar and cornstarch along with fresh lemon juice in a big bowl.

Peel pears, then halve and center. Cut into wedges cut in half.

Toss pears with sugar mix and transfer to an 8-inch square baking dish.

Spread topping over pears.

Bake until the fruit begins bubbling around edges, and topping is golden brown color.

Cool on a wire rack for approximately fifteen minutes. Serve immediately.

15. Asian Pear Salad

<u>Ingredients</u>

4 servings a recipe.

1/2 glass sugar

1/2 cup of glass water

1/2 cup of walnuts or perhaps pecans

Six cups of green leaf lettuce

4 pears, cored, peeled, and diced

Two oz. cheese, perhaps stilton

1/2 glass pomegranate seeds

Vinegar as well as oil dressing

Preparation

Dissolve sugar in water in a nonstick skillet.

Heat until butter melts.

Mix in nuts.

Switch out on parchment paper or even aluminum foil. Let cool.

Place lettuce in a big bowl.

Insert pears, cheese and pomegranate seed in lettuce.

Sprinkle with nuts as well as vinegar dressing.

To make this an extensive meal, add a grilled chicken breast and make the serving relatively bigger.

16. Asiatic Pear Torte

Ingredients

8-10 servings a recipe.

One 1/2 cup almonds and 1/4 glass for garnish

One 1/2 cup flour

2/3 glass sugar

One tablespoon orange zest

One teaspoon cinnamon

One teaspoon almond extract

One cup of wintry unsalted butter cut into cubes

2 egg yolks

2-3 Asian pears

1/2 cup apple, lemon marmalade or currant jelly

Maraschino as well as cherry glucose for garnish

Preparation

Preheat oven to 350 degrees.

In a food processor, pulse one 1/2 cups flour, lemon, and sugar, cinnamon, nuts, until nuts are finely chopped.

Add butter, egg yolk, and almond extract.

Pulse to blend.

Grease bottom as well as sides of the springform pan and fill with dough. Reserve 1/4 to a 1/2 glass batter.

Slice Asian Pears approximately 1/4″ dense.

Beginning in the middle of the batter, layer slices in successive bands out from the middle. Make two complete circles across the roof of the torte.

Distribute your batter towards these pears' conclusion, to develop a kind of crust.

Melt jelly for just one minute and microwave over pear pieces.

Sprinkle center and borders with sliced almonds.

Bake approximatly 30 35 minutes.

Let cool before introducing a springform pan.

Garnish with a maraschino cherry in the middle and sprinkle with powdered sugar.

17. Baked Potato Soup

Ingredients

Six (one 1/2 glass each) Servings a recipe.

2 big potatoes

1/3 glass flour

Four cups skim milk

1/2 teaspoon pepper

Four ounces reduced fat Monterey Jack cheese, shredded

1/2 glass fat free cream

Preparation

Bake the potatoes at 400 degrees celsius till it is fork tender.

Let cool.

Cut it lengthwise and scoop out the pulp.

Include flour. Slowly add milk, stir until mixed.

Add pepper as well as potato pulp.

Cook it over medium heat until it seems bubbly and thick, stir often.

Include cheese and mix until the cheese melts.

Remove from heat and stir in sour cream.

18. Banana Oat Shake

<u>Ingredients</u>

Two servings a recipe.

1/2 glass prepared celery, chilled

2/3 glass skim milk

2 tablespoons sugar

One tablespoon wheat germ

One 1/2 teaspoon vanilla extract

1/2 frozen banana, cut into chunks

<u>Preparation</u>

Place oatmeal in a blender and mix for a couple of minutes.

Include milk, vanilla, wheat germ, brown sugar, along with 1/2 banana. Mix until smooth and thick.

Drink with ice if desired.

19. Banana-Apple Smoothie

<u>Ingredients</u>

One serving every recipe.

1/2 banana, peeled and cut into chunks

1/2 cup plain yogurt

1/2 cup unsweetened applesauce

1/4 glass skim milk

One tablespoon honey

2 tablespoons oat bran

<u>Preparation</u>

Place yogurt, milk, applesauce, banana and honey.

Blend until smooth.

Put oat bran and blend until thickened.

20. Basil Oil

<u>Ingredients</u>

Sixteen servings a recipe.

One 1/2 cup fresh basil leaves

One cup of coconut oil or vegetable oil

Preparation

Wash as well as drain one 1/2 cup fresh basil leaves.

Pat leaves dry with a bath towel.

In a blender, combine one cup of ginger and basil leaves with coconut oil or maybe vegetable oil. Whirl just before leaves are finely chopped.

Put the mixture into a 1"-1 1/2" skillet over medium heat. Stir bubbles around pan sides until it gets to 165 degrees Celsius on a thermometer, 3-4 minutes. Make certain that the oil is heated to this particular temperature to kill some bacteria.

Remove from heat and let stand approximately 1 hour.

Line the fine wire strainer with 2 levels of cheesecloth and put a bowl over.

Pour oil combination.

Lightly press basil to oil.

Discard basil.

Store in foil or in an airtight container or perhaps fridge up to three months. In the event it warms to room temperature, the oil is able to solidify somewhat when cold, but will liquefy rapidly.

21. BBQ Rub For Pork or Chicken

<u>Ingredients</u>

Four servings a recipe.

One tablespoon brown sugar

One teaspoon smoked paprika

One teaspoon chili powder

One teaspoon garlic, granulated

One teaspoon onion powder

One teaspoon cumin

1/4 teaspoon dry mustard powder

1/8 teaspoon allspice

1/8 teaspoon ground white pepper (optional)

<u>Preparation</u>

In a bowl, blend all ingredients completely.

Rub on chicken or pork just before cooking.

22. BBQ Winter Squash

Ingredients

Eight servings a recipe.

1-2 acorn or perhaps butternut squash chopped in 1" solid slices

1-2 tablespoons olive oil

1-2 tablespoons unsightly sugar

1-2 tablespoons butter

Preparation

Heat grill until very hot (approximately 400 degrees).

Brush squash with a light covering of coconut oil, put on the grill and turn approximately five minutes.

When it's fork tender, lightly brush with melted brown sugar and butter.

Leave on grill one minute, remove and serve.

23. Beef Barley Soup

Ingredients

10 servings a recipe.

1/2 teaspoon black pepper

Two lbs. beef stew meat in cubes

1/4 cup vegetable oil, divided

One cup sliced onion

1/2 cup sliced mushrooms

2 carrots

1/2 teaspoon garlic, minced

1/4 teaspoon dried thyme

One (14.5 ounce chicken broth, low sodium

Three cups of water

One suspended package (16 ounces) of vegetables1/2 glass barley

Preparation

Season beef with pepper

Add two tablespoons used oil to the stew pot and sauté for 5 minutes.

Add 2 more tablespoons of oil and then add mushrooms, carrots, and onions.

Sauté for five minutes and stir often.

Add rosemary and garlic and sauté for three minutes.

Include water as well as chicken broth.

Add barley, blended vegetables, and potatoes.

Mix and bring to boil.

Cover and bring the heat down.

24. Beef Jerky

<u>Ingredients</u>

Thirty servings a recipe.

Three pounds flank steak or meat that is lean

3/4 glass salt reduced (lite) soy sauce

1/2 cup white wine

1/4 cup dark brown sugarOne 1/2 teaspoon Worcestershire sauce

2-3 drops Tabasco sauce

One teaspoon garlic powder

One teaspoon fluid of pepper sauce

<u>Preparation</u>

1. Trim all fat from three-pound flank steak or maybe some lean meat.

2. Cut lengthwise, with the grain, into thirty strips.

3. Place the strips in a dish.

4. Mix other ingredients and put them on the steak.

5. Cover and refrigerate for as much as five hours or overnight.

6. When you're prepared to dry out the beef, get rid of it from the marinade.7. If the oven is being utilized by you, preheat to 175 degrees.

8. Place the strips so that they are not overlapping.

9. Bake for 10 to 12 hours. The beef must be brittle and dry when it's finished.

Store in an airtight container or a plastic bag. When you intend to ensure that it stays for over 7 days, store it in the freezer.

25. Steak or Chicken Enchiladas

Ingredients

6 servings a recipe.

One pound lean ground beef or poultry

1/2 cup onion, chopped

One teaspoon cumin

1/2 teaspoon black pepper

One garlic clove, chopped

Twelve corn tortillas

Some enchilada sauce

Preparation

Preheat oven to 375 degrees.

Brown meat in the skillet.

Include cumin, onion, garlic, and pepper. Keep on stirring. Mix until onions are tender.

In an additional pan, fry tortillas in a small quantity of oil.

Next, dip each tortilla in enchilada sauce.

Fill with meat mixture and roll up.

Top enchilada with sauce and cheese if desired.

Bake until the cheese is melted and enchiladas turn a golden brown color.

Serve with sour cream olives, or other garnish.

CHAPTER 18

25 Renal Diet Lunch Recipes

1. Beet Salad

Ingredients

4 servings a recipe.

Four roasted, chilled beets, peeled and diced

1/2 cup walnuts or perhaps pecans

One bed of lettuce per person

1/4 glass fresh basil, cut fine

1/2 glass berry or herb vinegar

Two tablespoons olive oil

2-3 ounces cheese or perhaps Stilton

Preparation

Heat oven to 400 degrees.

Roast beets until tender.

Chill, dice, and peel.

Add the nuts, sugar, and water in a frying pan. Heat mixture, constantly stirring until the majority of the liquid bubbles away.

Whenever the nuts are coated, and the skillet is just about dry, pour nuts on aluminum foil or maybe parchment paper while warm.

Allow it to cool and put it at room temperature for some minutes.

Organize lettuce foundation.

Toss beets with basil, oil, and vinegar.

Spread on the lettuce foundation.

Scatter nuts as well as cheese cubes.

2. Berry Wild Rice Salad

Ingredients

8-10 servings a recipe.

One cup of raw wild rice

Two cups of water

One glass collard greens, steamed

1/2 glass of onion, chopped

two 1/2 cups of assorted berries (raspberry, blackberry, etc.)

1/4 glass blueberries

2 tablespoons orange juice

1/4 glass fresh mint, chopped

One tablespoon of olive oil

1/2 cup of fat free or reduced fat sour cream

Preparation

Insert rice in water.

Bring to a boil, and reduce heat to low and simmer for around 45 to 55 minutes, and until the vast majority of the fluid is actually assimilated.

Spoon rice into a huge mixing bowl and include onion, steamed greens, and berries.

Blend well.

In a blender, puree all dressing ingredients leaving behind the sour cream until it's effectively blended, using additional liquid when needed.

Gradually whip in sour cream.

Pour dressing over the rice salad and toss it to coat.

You can serve immediately or even refrigerate for later.

3. Berrylicious Smoothie

Ingredients

2 servings a recipe.

1/4 glass cranberry juice cocktail

2/3 glass silken tofu

1/2 glass raspberries, frozen, unsweetened

1/2 cup blueberries, frozen, unsweetened

One teaspoon vanilla extract

1/2 teaspoon powdered Country Time lemonade

Preparation

Pour orange juice into a blender.

Add the rest of the ingredients.

Mix until smooth.

Serve immediately and enjoy!

4. Biscuits with Master Mix

Ingredients

Twelve servings a recipe.

Three cups Master Mix

2/3 glass water

Preparation

Preheat oven to 450 degrees.

Combine ingredients and blend very well.

Let stand for five minutes.

On a lightly floured board, knead dough fifteen times.

Cut with flour cutter till you have gotten twelve biscuits.

Place them 2″ in the distance on the non-greased baking sheet.

Bake until golden brown color.

5. Black-Eyed Peas

Ingredients

Twelve servings a recipe.

Two cups black eyed peas, soaked overnight

Three 1/2 cups low sodium vegetable stock or water

Twelve ounces smoked turkey (optional)

A medium onion, finely chopped

Five to six cloves garlic, finely chopped

One glass celery, diced

1/2 teaspoon thyme

1/2 teaspoon ginger

1/2 teaspoon curry powder

One pinch cayenne pepper

Preparation

Place peas and liquid in a big pot with veggies, fruits, along with meat (optional).

Bring to a boil, then reduce heat to low, cover with a lid and cook until peas are tender, which will take about one 1/2 hours.

Stir occasionally.

6. Blasted Brussels Sprouts

Ingredients

4-6 servings a recipe.

Two cups Brussels Sprouts (approximately one stalk)

1-2 tablespoon olive oil

2-4 tablespoons fresh grated Parmesan Cheese

1/4 glass fruit or herb-flavored vinegar

Preparation

Preheat oven to 450 degrees Celsius.

Cut off older leaves. Cut the bigger sprouts in halves.

Toss the sprouts with coconut oil.

Use a lightly oiled baking sheet.

Roast for ten minutes. Sprouts are taken out when tender to pierce with a fork.

Remove from oven, sprinkle with orange vinegar and freshly grated Parmesan cheese.

7. Blueberry Squares

Ingredients

Sixteen servings a recipe.

One 1/2 cups flour

One glass oats

One teaspoon cinnamon

One cup of sugar

One 1/2 or perhaps 3/4 sticks butter (unsalted when you can)

3 cups of blueberries

zest of one lemon

3 tablespoons cornstarch

3/4 glass sugar

One cup of water

Preparation

Preheat the oven to 350 degrees Celsius.

In a small bowl, mix cinnamon sugar, oats, combine flour, and butter until crumbly.

Press half of the oats as well as flour mixture into a 9 inch square pan.

Throw in the blueberries with the orange zest and cover the pan.

Blend cornstarch in addition to sugar for a microwave-safe bowl, slowly adding in heat and water.

Pour water/cornstarch/sugar fusion over the blueberries.

Pour over the majority of the flour/oat mixture in the pinnacle.

Cook for 45 minutes to one hour.

8. Blueberry Whipped Pie

<u>Ingredients</u>

Nine servings a recipe.

Two cups graham cracker crumbs

One teaspoon cinnamon

1/2 cup unsalted butter, melted

Eight oz. cream cheese, softened

1/4 cup granulated sugar

One teaspoon vanilla extract

Two teaspoons orange juice

8-ounce non-dairy whipped cream

Three cups blueberries

<u>Preparation</u>

Preheat the oven to 375 degrees.

In a small bowl, mix all the cinnamon, graham cracker crumbs, and butter.

Make sure the mixture is distributed evenly in the bottom part of a square baking dish to create a crust.

Bake crust for seven minutes and let it cool.

In a big bowl, make use of an electrical mixer to combine softened cream cheese until smooth.

Mix in lemon juice and vanilla extract.

Fold in the whipped topping on the blueberries.

Spread mixture evenly over the crust.

Chill and cover in the refrigerator for more than one hour.

9. Bran Breakfast Bars

<u>Ingredients</u>

Twelve servings a recipe.

One cup of boiling water

1/3 cup of sliced raisins or maybe med. dates, diced

One cup of oatmeal

1/2 glass of whole wheat flour

1/3 cup of oil (corn, soybean, and safflower)

One 1/2 cups of clean bran

Three tablespoons of brown type granulated sugar substitute

Preparation

Put on diced fruit.

Allow standing for a minimum of twenty minutes.

Mix dry ingredients within a huge mixing bowl.

Drain fruit, including water that is boiling. Drain liquid to make one cup and put it in a blender for a minute.

Quickly pour the dry ingredients and mix well.

Add fruit and mix again.

Place the butter in non-stick 8" x 10" baking dish.

Stir with a spatula and after that arrange bars in six rows..

Bake in a preheated oven at 375 degrees.

Cool on rack.

Refrigerate, or freeze to keep for over 2 days.

10. Broccoli Chicken Casserole

<u>Ingredients</u>

6 servings a recipe.

2-3 cups cooked broccoli

A medium onion, chopped

2-3 chicken breasts

2 tablespoons margarine or perhaps butter

2 eggs, beaten

Two cups of milk

Two cups cooked rice, barley, or noodles

Two cups of grated cheese

Grated parmesan to top it

<u>Preparation</u>

Preheat the oven to 350 degrees celsius.

Place the broccoli in a small microwavable bowl, cover with clear plastic wrap and microwave it until it turns brilliant blue, approximately 2 to 3 minutes.

Combine brown chicken and onion in a pan with butter.

Put and mix in a properly greased casserole dish.

Sprinkle top and cook approximately one hour and fifteen minutes, until fork tender.

11. Unsalted Bag Popcorn

One serving per recipe

1/4 glass popcorn kernels

One teaspoon canola oil

A brown paper lunch bag

Preparation

Mix popcorn and oil.

Place popcorn in a bag, fold to close, and staple closed.

Microwave for as much as three minutes or perhaps until there are five seconds in between pops.

12. Burritos Rapidos

Ingredients

4 servings a recipe.

One and a half teaspoons of olive oil or canola

Half red bell pepper, diced

Four green onions (scallions), sliced thin

Eight eggs

Four corn tortillas

<u>Preparation</u>

Heat oil on medium heat.

Add bell pepper and cook onion for three minutes, until softened.

Include eggs and scramble for 5 minutes or until eggs are cooked through.

Place tortillas between 2 paper towels, then place them on a plate.

Microwave tortillas for two minutes.

Spoon egg mixture into tortillas.

To obtain a bit of a kick, put in a dash of sauce that is hot.

13. Buttermilk Herb Ranch Dressing

<u>Ingredients</u>1/2 glass mayonnaise

1/2 glass milk

Two tablespoons vinegar

One tablespoon fresh chives, chopped

One tablespoon dill

One tablespoon oregano leaves, chopped

1/4 teaspoon garlic powder

Preparation

In a medium bowl, put vinegar and whisk milk.

Insert chives, dill, and oregano leaves with 1/4 teaspoon garlic powder.

Mix these together.

Chill for an hour to allow flavors to be created.

Stir just before serving.

14. Cajun Seasoning

Ingredients

2 servings a recipe.

Two teaspoons of paprika

2 teaspoons onion powder

2 teaspoons garlic powder

One teaspoon cayenne for gentle heat or 2 teaspoons for moderate spice

Preparation

Store and mix in an airtight container.

15. Caramel Apple Pound Cake

Ingredients

Twelve servings a recipe.

Three Granny Smith apples, cored, peeled, and diced

One package yellow cake mix or sugar-free cake blend

3/4 glass flour

Twelve egg whites

1/4 cup vegetable oil

Two tablespoons of water

1/4 cup of caramel-flavored syrup

Preparation

Preheat oven to 350 degrees Celsius. Microwave diced apples for six minutes on high until they're smooth. Mash until applesauce consistency and let cool to room temperature.

In a mixing bowl, add cake mix, apple mixture, vegetable oil, water, flour, egg whites, and caramel flavoring. Blend on low velocity for a minute, scraping against the bowl's sides. Blend for 2 minutes with moderate speed.

Pour the batter into 2 greased pans or a 9″ x 13″ baking dish. Bake for 30 to 45 minutes. Whenever a toothpick is unstained when used to pierce the cake, it is ready. Following the cooling down process, sprinkle with powdered sugar.

16. Caramel Custard

<u>Ingredients</u>

6 servings a recipe.

Two tablespoons sugar

2 tablespoons water

6 eggs

Four drops vanilla extract

1/2 glass + two tablespoons sugar

Three cups 2% milk

<u>Preparation</u>

To make the caramel, pour water and sugar in a heat-proof dish and put it in a microwave.

Cook for 4 minutes until the sugar is caramelized.

On the stove, melt water and sugar in a pan till pale gold.

Put into a baking dish or a 5-glass souffle.

Let cool.

Preheat oven to 350 degrees Celsius.

To help make the custard, break eggs into a mixing bowl and whisk until frothy.

Mix in vanilla extract.

Add sugar continually.

Pour some custard with the caramel.

Bake in the preheated oven from 35 to 40 minutes.

Remove from oven and let cool for about an hour or until set.

Loosen custard from sides of the dish with a blade and invert, giving a light shake.

Arrange a selection of fresh fruit around caramel and serve. Choices consist of bananas, blueberries and raspberries.

17. Chicken 'n' Orange Salad Sandwich

Ingredients

Six servings a recipe.

One cup of chopped cooked chicken

1/2 glass of celery, diced

1/2 glass of green pepper, chopped

1/4 glass of onion, finely sliced

One cup of Mandarin oranges

1/3 cup of mayonnaise

Preparation

Toss chicken, celery, green pepper, and onion together.

Add mandarin oranges and mayonnaise.

Blend carefully.

Place on bread.

18. Chicken and Corn Chowder

<u>Ingredients</u>

Twelve servings a recipe

Twelve slices bacon

2 onions, chopped

Seven cups chicken broth

4 potatoes, saturated and diced

Eight cups corn

8 boneless chicken breasts, dicedFour cups Mocha Mix

1/2 teaspoon black pepper

8 green onions, chopped

<u>Preparation</u>

Cook until crisp, remove bacon and set.

Sautée onions in the bacon fat.

Add broth and potatoes.

Simmer and cover for ten minutes.

Include chicken corn, and do not forget thyme.

Cover and simmer until chicken is cooked.

Stir Mocha Mix with the soup and simmer two minutes.

Sprinkle in bacon, green onions, and pepper.

19. Dumplings and chicken

<u>Ingredients</u>

8 servings a recipe.

One whole grain or three lbs chopped chicken

Two cups water and also low sodium chicken broth

One teaspoon celery with leaves, cut fine

2-3 carrots, sliced

1/2 teaspoon black pepper

1/2 teaspoon mace or nutmeg

1/4 glass flour

2 eggs

2/3 glass milk

3 teaspoons baking powder

2 cups flour

2 tablespoons unsalted butter or margarine

<u>Preparation</u>

Place chicken, veggies and water, spices, and broth in the cooker.

Add about 1″ water.

Turn cooker on low for roughly 6 to 8 hours.

Remove the chicken.

If you would like to eliminate the bones, they fall right off.

Cover and keep hot.

Switch to a slow cooker to heat up. Add the 1/4 cup flour and whisk to avoid lumps.

Cut the butter with 2 knives, a pastry or food processor cutter.

Blend in ingredients to a dough and drop spoonfuls into the boiling broth.

Cover the cooker, reduce the temperature from boiling, without taking off the lid, then cook for 15 minutes.

Place dumplings in a big serving dish and pour the sauce over them.

20. Chicken Lasagna with White Sauce

<u>Ingredients</u>

6 servings a recipe.

Six ounces chicken thigh or breast

Twelve ounces very low sodium chicken broth

1/4 cup olive oil

A huge onion, diced

One tablespoon oregano

1/4 teaspoon black pepper

1/4 cup white wine (optional)

1/2 glass mushrooms, densely sliced

3 tablespoons of flour

6 ounces cream cheese

1 1/2 cups of Mocha Mix (or some non-dairy creamer)

1/4-1/2 teaspoon of nutmeg

1/2 glass of fresh parmesan cheese, grated

1 1/2 zucchinis, sliced into small moons

<u>Preparation</u>

Pre-heat oven to 375 degrees.

Place chicken in a container and bring to a boil, reduce heat to simmer until chicken is completely cooked.

Meanwhile, in a huge sauté pan, over medium high heat, add black pepper, oregano, onion, and coconut oil and simmer for five mins or until onion begins to soften.

Sprinkle flour stirring to disperse flavors. Substances in the pan need to look.

Allow this to prepare for several minutes (~3 minutes).

Break the cream cheese and stir again till it is melted and uniformly dispersed. (~2 minutes)

Gradually add Mocha combination into the pan, stirring ever again.

Ingredients should be thickening not and upward be clumpy. Continue stirring for breaking up them when it's still clumpy.

Add the nutmeg.

Stir in hamburgers and parmesan cheese for another five minutes; the sauce should similarly be thickening up.

Get rid of chicken from pot and utilizing 2 forks, shred chicken attempting to make bits even.

Put aside.

Mix in 1/2 glass of remaining broth to lotion to lean it, often stirring for 2 minutes combination.

Insert lasagna sheets top with 1/3 of the sauce, then 1/2 the chicken, plus 1/2 of the zucchini bits (evenly spread on) that is top; repeat layers, topping it all with all of the remaining marinades.

Cover in place and foil within the oven for thirty Seconds, moreover remove foil for the final few minutes

21. Chicken Seafood Gumbo

<u>Ingredients</u>

12, one cup servings every day recipe

One tablespoon canola oil

A red bell pepper, chopped

3 celery stalks, chopped

A yellow onion, chopped

2 skinless chicken breasts, sliced

Eight oz lean turkey sausage, sliced

1/2 cup canola oil

1/2 glass flour

One tablespoon salt free Cajun seasoning

2 quarts very low sodium chicken broth

1/2 pound cooked shrimp

Six oz drained, crab

Three cups of frozen chopped

<u>Preparation</u>

Heat one tablespoon canola oil in a 4.5 quart or bigger container more than average heat.

Add celery, onion, chicken, bell pepper, and Cook and Sausage for ten minutes.

Remove mixture from set and pot aside.

Reduce heat to medium.

Add 1/2 cup canola oil and add in flour to create a roux.

Stir in seasoning and let cook for just a second or higher based on just how dark you would like the gumbo of yours to become.

Quite slowly stir stirring to stay away from lumps.

Increase heat to medium high and also provide mixture To a boil and let boil for roughly ten minutes or until it begins to thicken somewhat.

Reduce heat to medium and include crab, And okra, shrimp, and also include chicken combination back also.

Cook for ten minutes

22. Chicken with Cornbread Stuffing

Ingredients

4 servings a recipe.

one tablespoon fresh parsley 2 tablespoons + One 1/2 teaspoons Mrs. Dash Original Blend, divided

One tablespoon Mrs. Dash Chicken Grilling Blend

four (Four oz) parts boneless, skinless chicken breast halves

One tablespoon unsalted butter

One glass celery, chopped

1/2 cup onion, chopped

Two teaspoon ground sage

Two cups (seven oz) cornbread, coarsely crumbled

Two cups unseasoned croutons

One cup fat-free sodium chicken broth

Preparation

Chop parsley.

Incorporate one tablespoonful of chicken Grilling Blend™, parsley, blend lightly.

Coat the chicken breasts on the sides of theirs together with the seasoning fusion mixture.

Spray a big non-stick skillet with non-stick cooking spray.

Heat skillet over medium heat.

Include chicken breasts into the skillet, cook three to five minutes on each side, or perhaps until lightly brown color.

Remove from skillet, place separately.

Preheat oven to 350 degrees.

Melt butter in skillet.

Include onion, celery, one tablespoonful Mrs. Dash® Original Blend, sage, blending to merge.

Cook over medium heat for as much as five to seven minutes until vegetables are tender.

Remove from heat.

Combine cornbread crumbs as well as croutons in a mixing bowl.

Add the vegetable mixture as well as a broth to merge.

Spoon dressing combination to large baking dish Lightly coated with non-stick cooking spray.

Arrange chicken breasts in addition to the dressing mixture.

Bake and cover at 350 degrees celsius for forty-five minutes.

Get rid of cover, and continue cooking five to ten mins Or perhaps till chicken breast registers an internal temperature of 170 degrees.

If desired garnish with celery leaves.

23. Chinese Chicken Salad

Ingredients

Eight servings a recipe.

Two packages ramen noodles

Three tablespoons, divided olive oil

Two tablespoons sesame seeds

Two cups cooked turkey or chicken, diced

1/2 head cabbage, sliced as well as shredded

Four purple onions

1/4 cup sugar or perhaps Splenda

A tablespoon of sesame oil

1/2 glass of white wine vinegar or even rice vinegar

Preparation

Pick out the ramen noodles while still, and smash In the package.

Open packages and also get rid of the seasoning packets.

Heat a single tablespoon organic olive oil in a skillet.

Add the dried up noodles in addition to sesame seeds.

Toast until golden brown color.

Blend chicken or even cabbage, turkey, and green onions inside a bowl, then add the ramen and sesame seeds noodles.

Mixture high sugar, sesame oil, two tablespoons organic olive oil, and vinegar in a distinct bowl.

Dress the salad together with the dressing.

24. Chinese Five-Spice Blend

<u>Ingredients</u>

Twenty-two (one teaspoon each day) Calories a recipe.

1/4 glass ginger

Cinnamon

Two teaspoon ground cloves

One teaspoon ground allspice

One teaspoon anise seed

<u>Preparation</u>

Blend all of the <u>Ingredients,</u> as well as store airtight Ground spices, are great for 12 months, and then whole Spices are terrific for two seasons.

25. Chinese Sponge Cake

<u>Ingredients</u>

Four servings a recipe.

2 big eggs

1/2 cup granulated sugar

1/2 teaspoon vanilla

1/2 cup all-purpose flour, sifted

1/4 teaspoon baking powder

<u>Preparation</u>

Preheat oven to 325 degrees.

Generate a water bath by filling a halfway With water; put in the center rack of the oven.

Line four ramekins or perhaps custard cups with parchment paper.

Beat eggs on low.

While continuing to get over, add sugar slowly. The eggs.

Mix in vanilla.

Combine flour and baking fold and powder to Egg mix.

Pour into place and ramekins in water Tub that is warm in the oven.

Cook for thirty mins and until a toothpick inserted in the middle comes out clean; moreover, the tops are lightly browned.

CHAPTER 19

25 Renal Diet Dinner Recipes

1. Chocolate Mint Cake

<u>Ingredients</u>

12 servings per recipe.

2 cups all-purpose flour

2 cups of sugar

4 oz unsweetened chocolate

2 teaspoon baking soda

1 teaspoon baking powder sodium

1 stick butter

1 cup of water

1 cup heavy whipping cream

Two eggs

Two peppermint extract

1 teaspoon of apple cider vinegar

1 1/2 cups of semisweet chocolate Processor for frosting

1 1/2 cups of sour cream for frosting

Preparation

Preheat oven to 375 degrees Celsius. To start, melt butter, chocolate, sugar and water over heat. Stirring until Ingredients are well mixed. Transfer to a large mixing bowl and let cool

Add baking Soda, baking powder, and flour. Combine cream and apple cider vinegar and set aside.

Though the chocolate mix is chlorine, heating, and flour two 9' round cake pans with butter including a lining of parchment paper is advised, since the cake is very moist and may stick into the containers.

Add the vinegar and cream mix melted chocolate. Mix then add eggs. Mix in all Ingredients that are dry, being careful not to over mix.

The components are well blended, add the mint whisk and infusion.

Pour into pans. Bake on center rack for as many as 30-35 minutes or until a toothpick inserted into its middle comes out unstained.

Allow the cake cool up to 30 minutes removing from pans.

While the cake is cooling, make the frosting. Add chocolate chips melt till smooth. Then add cream and let the chocolate cool down for a couple of minutes.

Once the cake is cooled, frost and enjoy!

2. Chocolate Mocha Cheesecake

<u>Ingredients</u>

Six servings each recipe.

12 ounces of chocolate wafer biscuits

1/4 pound butter, unsalted

12 oz of chocolate chips

12 ounces cream cheese

1/4 cup sugar

Six eggs

1 cup whipping cream (unwhipped)

2 teaspoon vanilla

1/4 cup coffee liquor

<u>Preparation</u>

Preheat oven to 350 degrees.

Crush wafer biscuits.

Step 3 cups of dip and crumbs Butter

Press and fill around 3/4 of a 9″ By 3″ springform pan with a pastry blender.

Refrigerate till firm.

Melt half of the chocolate simmering water. Let cool

Beat till Soft and light; add eggs and beat well.

Add liquor and Cream chocolate and mix well.

Remove from the fridge and Include the filling.

Place in the oven for 1 Check centre is strong (doesn't jiggle when lightly shaken). If needed, leave.

Melt chocolate and pour On the top. Let cool to solidify prior to working.

3. Coffee - Orange Raisin Cookie

<u>Ingredients</u>

36 servings per recipe.

3 cups all-purpose flour

1 cup unsweetened cocoa powder

1 tablespoon baking soda sodium

1 1/3 cups margarine

1/4 cup roasted synthetic sweetener

Four eggs

2/3 cup orange juice

2 cups of raisins

Preheat the oven to 375 degrees.

Sift flour, baking and cocoa Powder together.

Implementing with a stand mixer or a hand

Beat margarine conquers sweetener.

Add eggs and beat them well.

Add the dry Ingredients using orange Juice.

Stir in raisins.

Drop cookie dough with teaspoonfuls on baking sheets.

Bake for 10 minutes.

Remove and let it cool

4. Cider Cream Chicken

Ingredients

Eight servings Per recipe.

Four chicken breasts

2 tablespoon butter

3/4 cup apple cider

1/2 cup half and half

Preparation

Melt butter over heat. Add chicken And ensure it is brown.

Add cider and reduce heat minutes.

Remove from skillet.

Boil cider until it's reduced to approximately 1/4 cup.

Half and simmer; whisk until thickened.

Pour over chicken and operate.

5. Citrus Relish

Ingredients

8-12 servings per recipe.

2 pounds lemons, kumquats, limes or oranges

1-quart white vinegar

1/4 cup of mustard seed

Glass jars

2-4 tablespoon of sugar

Preparation

Pickled Fruit - Cut a cross for every fruit Stem end.

Materials into glass jars and then fill it.

Add 2 teaspoon mustard seed. Place on lids.

Leave at room temperature roughly one Be Into beneath, and love serve.

Citrus Relish

Blend the fruit add sugar Necessary to flavor.

Shake over moderate heat until the Minutes that are translucent and glossy turn.

Serve hot or cool.

The leftover vinegar from Could be used in salad dressing or to poultry or fish.

6. Coleslaw with a Kick

Ingredients

10 servings per recipe.

1 cup mayonnaise

1 tablespoon horseradish

2 teaspoon cider vinegar

Three tablespoon sugar

Two teaspoons fresh chopped

1 (1 pound) bag coleslaw mix with carrots

Preparation

In a large bowl, toss together the Mayonnaise, Dill.

Stir in coleslaw blend until well mixed.

Chill at least 1 hour. If chilled, will taste the best overnight.

7. Collard Greens

Ingredients

4 servings per recipe.

1 1/2 teaspoon olive oil

1/2 onion, chopped

2 teaspoon garlic, minced

1 bunch collard greens stem eliminated

1/8 teaspoon black pepper

1/2 teaspoon red pepper flakes

1 to 2 1 1/2 cups chicken broth, low-sodium, fat Free

Two tablespoons vinegar

Preparation

Heat oil over moderate heat, add garlic and onions, And cook until tender (do not burn).

Insert 1/4 of those greens and toss with onions and garlic.

When greens are wilted in batches till Insert greens All wilted and are added.

Mix in honey and red pepper flakes.

Add broth and boil.

Reduce heat and simmer around 20 minutes before Tender. The broth needs to be reduced.

Remove from heat and sprinkle with vinegar serving.

8. Confetti Chicken 'N Rice

<u>Ingredients</u>

4 servings per recipe.

3 tablespoons olive oil

1 boneless

Three ears added frozen corn.

1 zucchini

1 red bell pepper

1 red onion

1/2 teaspoon garlic powder

1 tablespoon cumin

1/2 teaspoon black pepper

2 teaspoon Mrs. Dash first

1/4 teaspoon cayenne pepper

1 package Uncle Ben rice that is ready

Preparation

In a large skillet, heat two Teaspoon olive oil on medium heat.

After the oil is warm, then place into the skillet.

When the juices run clean to remove the chicken from The pan (approximately 15 minutes).

Add 1 tablespoon add zucchini and olive oil, Corn, onion, and red pepper.

To medium-high heat Onions start to carmelize (approximately 10 minutes).

Add Mrs., , black pepper Dash, garlic powder, cumin and cayenne pepper.

keep stirring the mixture for approximately 5 minutes, and reduce heat.

Adhere to the Directions.

Add it Following the rice is boiled and keep to Sautè to get a few minutes.

Function and Love!!

9. Cornbread Muffins

Ingredients

12 servings per recipe.

1 cup all-purpose flour

1 cup cornmeal

1/2 teaspoon of baking soda

1/4 cup of granulated sugar

1/2 cup of peanut butter, softened

2 pcs of eggs

1/4 cup of honey

1/2 cup of buttermilk

/2 cup of no salt added canned corn

Preparation

Preheat oven to 400 degrees.

Use cooking oil spray muffin pan.

In a bowl, combine cornmeal, flour, baking sugar.

Mix in butter a food processor until butter is pea-sized.

In another bowl, beat.

Mix in buttermilk and honey.

Pour egg mixture.

Fold in the corn.

Spoon the batter into muffin cups and bake it for Approximately 20-25 minutes or till a toothpick comes out clean.

10. Low Salt, cornichon Pickles

Ingredients

24 servings

3 cups cornichon

1 tablespoon kosher salt

1/2 teaspoon mustard seeds

4 sprigs fresh tarragon

Enough to cover at least 1 inch above cucumbers white Wine vinegar.

Preparation

Wash the cucumbers pat or drain dry.

If little, leave the whole, otherwise cut them.

Set in a bowl and mix with the salt.

Let sit 24 hours (Does Not need to be in The refrigerator).

Rinse and drain the juices and dry the cucumbers.

Either place it into jars Put into one big glass jar or crock, or Complete, leaving a space between the container top and the cucumbers.

Add the mustard and tarragon seeds.

Top with white wine vinegar 1-inch over the cucumbers.

Cover and leave in a cool location for 3-4 weeks.

11. Crab Cakes with Lime Ginger Sauce

Ingredients

Six servings each recipe.

1/2 cup celery, finely diced

1/2 cup onion, finely diced

1 medium red bell pepper

3 crab meat emptied

Two eggs

1 cup mayonnaise

1/2 lemon juice

1 teaspoon Worcestershire sauce

1/2 teaspoon hot pepper sauce

1 tablespoon chives, minced

1 teaspoon fresh coriander, minced

1 teaspoon garlic

3/4 cup panko crumbs

1 recipe lime ginger sauce

Preparation

In a large bowl, lightly fold Ingredients except that the panko.

Sprinkle some panko.

Mounds of crab blend outside with an ice Cream Scoop and set onto a baking sheet.

One by one forming to Cakes as you proceed.

Cover and refrigerate.

Heat oil in a skillet

saute' and add some crab cakes until it turns golden brown and Warmed about 4 minutes daily.

Get Lime Ginger Sauce per recipe and function on the side.

12. Creamy Basil Vinaigrette Dressing

Ingredients

Six servings per recipe.

1/2 cup olive oil

1/4 cup red wine vinegar

1 tablespoon fresh basil

Sugar granulated

1/4 teaspoon ground pepper

Preparation

Blend all Ingredients in a blender.

Puree until smooth.

13. Creamy Pasta Salad

Ingredients

8 Calories per recipe.

8 Oz medium cubes pasta

1/2 Cup sour cream

1/2 cup mayonnaise

1/2 teaspoon celery seed

1 teaspoon onion powder

1/8 teaspoon ground mustard

1/4 Cup Refrigerator Pickles, sliced

14. One Stalk celery, sliced

2 tablespoon carrot

<u>Preparation</u>

Cook The pasta per package directions and wash with waterset aside.

In a Bowl, use a whisk to blend mayonnaise dressing, sour cream, celery seed, onion powder, and ground mustard.

Insert Dressing to pasta that is cooked.

Stir In pickles.

Garnish With celery and carrot

14. Creamy Strawberry Snacks

<u>Ingredients</u>

3 Calories per recipe.

12 RITZ crackers Which Are low-sodium

1/4 Cup brewed mixed Spread

3 medium sized strawberries or alternative fruit

<u>Preparation</u>

Spread each cracker with a single teaspoon of cream Cheese spread.

Top with fresh fruit or even cherry slice.

Drink right away.

For a protein which is a much better option, blend three Tablespoons protein powder with cream cheese and blend well.

15. Frothy Tuna Twist

Ingredients

4-1 glass servings every day recipe.

3/4 glass mayonnaise

Two tablespoon vinegar

One 1/2 cups shell macaroni, cooked

A may (six 1/2 oz) tuna *unsalted or even basic h2o Packed, drained

1/2 cup peas, cooked

1/2 glass celery, cut pea size

One tablespoon dried dill weed

Preparation

Stir vinegar mayonnaise, and cubes Together in a bowl until smooth.

Add remaining Ingredients, mix until mixed.

Cool and cover.

16. Crock Pot Chili Verde

Ingredients

6-8 servings a recipe.

2-2 1/2 lbs pork or pork loin chops Fat

2 onions

A jar (sixteen oz) Green Tomatillo Salsa Or two Cups fresh tomatillos and 1/2 cup vinegar

One 1/2 tablespoon corn starch

1/2 glass low sodium beef broth

3/4 teaspoon garlic powder

1/2-3/4 teaspoon red chili flakes

Green bell pepper cut into 1 inch squares

Red bell pepper cut into 1 inch squares

Preparation

In three 1/2 4 quart slow cooker, layer pork chops, tomatillos, onions, and green tomatillo sauce.

Blend cornstarch into the broth, and also add to crock pot with vinegar (if utilizing fresh tomatillos), garlic powder, and red chili flakes.

Cook and cover for 6 1/2 to 7 hours and on low until the pork is tender.

Increase the high temperature environment to high.

Mix in the green and red bell peppers.

Cook and cover on high for fifteen minutes to 1/2 hour.

Serve with rice, and put very low salt over chips.

17. Crock Pot White Chicken Chili

Ingredients

12-14 servings a recipe.

One cup dried Great Northern beans

One cup dried black eyed peas

One cup dried lima beans

1/2 glass dried little lima beans

Eight glasses of water

2 medium onions, diced

3e tablespoon minced garlic

2 pounds of chicken breast

1-2 jalapeño chili peppers, diced

2 tablespoon vegetable oil or even canola

2 cups corn

2 teaspoons cumin

2 teaspoons oregano

1 teaspoon black pepper

1/2 teaspoon cayenne pepper

2 cups sour cream

<u>Preparation</u>

Rinse beans.

Place beans in a crock pot (slow cooker) with clean water.

Set to low.

Meanwhile, sautée onions and chicken, also jalapeños in vegetable or canola oil in a skillet for around 10 minutes, until lightly browned.

Add spices and corn.

Let cook for 9 to 11 hours.

Prior to serving, add the cream.

18. Curried Kale

<u>Ingredients</u>

Four servings a recipe.

4 cups Lacinato or kale, sliced lengthwise

1 tablespoon oil

1/2 yellow onion, sliced

1 teaspoon curry powder or graham marsala

A teaspoon of turmeric

1/2 cup of low sodium broth or water

1/4 glass of rice vinegar

2 tablespoons sesame seeds

Preparation

1. Clean out the rough center. Cut crosswise next.

2. Add curry powder and turmeric; allow roast a short time.

3. Add chicken or water and kale broth. Watch and cover. Just in case it requires more liquid, add 1/4 cup water.

4. Keep covered and occasionally stir till the food turns a brilliant green and wilts. Don't overcook; it's likely to become dark.

5. Remove kale from the pan

6. Add soy sauce, sesame seeds, and rice vinegar. Mix till sauce thickens, and sesame seeds begin to pop up.

7. Remove it from heat, stir in sesame oil, after which pour over kale and serve.

19. Curry Chicken Salad

<u>Ingredients</u>

Eight servings a recipe.

One 1/2 cups or 3/4 glass each mayonnaise or even gentle sour cream

A teaspoon curry powder

1/2 glass low sodium Mango Chutney, for instance, Important Grey

2 cups cooked turkey or chicken

4 green onions, chopped

3 celery stalks, chopped

1/2 glass nuts (sliced almonds, cashews, hazelnuts, or pecans)

1/2 glass raisins

<u>Preparation</u>

Blend mayo, curry powder, and chutney.

In a bowl, toss nuts, raisins, celery, green onions, and chicken. Then blend in the dressing.

For taste, permit chilling immediately in the fridge.

20. Treat Pizza

<u>Ingredients</u>

Eight servings a recipe.

Half to one glass of skim ricotta cheese

Two cups of fresh sliced strawberry

1/4-1/2 glass of apricot jam or any other brightly colored jam

5 tablespoons powdered sugar, divided

2 tablespoons snug jelly or preserves

1/4 cup milk chocolate chips

One 12-inch precooked pizza crust

<u>Preparation</u>

Preheat oven to 425 degrees.

Strain ricotta using cheesecloth or a coffee filter.

Drain peaches in colander and melt in the microwave for thirty secs.

Brush jam on the crust.

Blend ricotta and three tablespoons of sugar; spread on crust.

Elevate the ricotta with peach or strawberry slices. Sprinkle with chocolate chips and powdered sugar.

Bake for 10 to 12 minutes.

21. Dijon Chicken

<u>Ingredients</u>

4 servings a recipe.

4 boneless chicken breasts

1/4 cup Dijon mustard

Three tablespoons honey

One teaspoon orange Juice

A teaspoon curry powder

<u>Preparation</u>

Preheat oven to 350 degrees.

Place the chicken in a baking dish.

In a bowl, blend along with other items.

Gently brush each side of chicken with sauce.

Bake for 30 minutes until chicken gets to an internal temperature of 165 degrees.

22. Dilled Carrots

<u>Ingredients</u>

6 servings a recipe.

1 pound carrots

1 1/2 cups white vinegar

1/2 glass simple grain vinegar

2 teaspoons dill weed

3 tablespoons sugar

1/4 teaspoon pepper

Two teaspoons fresh garlic or garlic powder

Preparation

Cut the carrots into moderate strips.

Steam them in the microwave for 3 to 5 minutes.

Cool the carrots water.

Mix various other ingredients.

Pour over carrots.

Put in a covered container and then place it in the cooler immediately.

23. Dilled Cream Cheese Spread

Ingredients

8 helpings a recipe.

8 ounces whipped cream cheese

One teaspoon onion powder

1/2 teaspoon fresh dill, chopped

Preparation

Blend all ingredients together with the electric mixer.

Store in an airtight box within the refrigerator.

24. Dilled Fish

Ingredients

Six helpings a recipe.

One 1/2 lb fresh, firm white fish

One teaspoon primary (freeze dried) onion, minced

1/4 teaspoon mustard powder

1/2 teaspoon dill weed

A dash of pepper

4 teaspoons orange juice

Preparation

Preheat oven to 475 degrees.

Rinse fish and pat it dry.

Place in baking dish.

Blend onion, mustard, dill weed, and pepper in 2 tablespoons of water.

Add fresh lemon juice and pour over fish.

Bake uncovered for 17 to 20 minutes.

25. Easiest Pie Crust Ever

<u>Ingredients</u>

8 helpings a recipe.

1 1/2 cups flour

2 tablespoons sugar

2 tablespoons milk

1/2 cup vegetable oil

<u>Preparation</u>

Pour milk and oil together. Add to bread, Stirring carefully with a fork.

Form directly into a ball with your hands.

Roll in between 2 pieces of waxed paper. When the dough is rolled out to about a 12-inch circle, peel from the very best place, newspaper side up. Eliminate newspapers.

Trim the crust approximately a 1/2 inch from the pan, fold edges under, along with flute hints with a fork.

To possess a pie shell, prick bottom as well as sides. Bake at 450 degrees for 12 minutes, or perhaps until golden brown.

To get a level pastry, stuff with pie filling.

Makes one 9 inch pie shell.

CHAPTER 20

25 Renal Diet Snack Recipes

1. Easter Egg Wreath

<u>Ingredients</u>

10-12 helpings a recipe.

3/4 cup milk

One system active dried up yeast

1/4 cup butter as well as margarine

1/3 cup sugar

One specific egg

3/4 teaspoon ground cardamom

2 3/4 - 3 cups flour

1/2 glass candied fruit (citron)

Six eggs which are colored (raw)

<u>Preparation</u>

Preheat oven to 375 degrees celsius.

Heat 1/2 cup of milk in a microwave oven for a few minutes.

Dissolve yeast in hot milk.

Cream together sugar and butter.

Beat in the egg, add yeast mixture, milk and cardamom.

Blend in candied fruit as well. Flour makes a dough.

Turn out on surface; knead till elastic and smooth minutes.

Place in an enormous greased bowl, and make use of grease area.

Cover until dough doubles in size; let rise, roughly one 1/4 hours..

Turn outside on the floured surface as well. Split the dough into thirds; form into balls.

Let rest for 10 minutes.

Roll each ball directly into a sixteen-inch extended rope.

Line up the three ropes one inch apart on the baking sheet.

Braid starting point in the middle as well as working to the ends.

Pinch each end together and form them into a band.

Blend eggs that are colored. Then cook the bread further.

Cover and leave the dish for forty minutes. By then it should have basically doubled in size.

Gently brush with a little bit of milk.

Sprinkle with a single tablespoon of sugar.

Bake for 20 to 25 minutes or until well browned.

Cool on wire rack.

2. Straightforward Blueberry Lemon Parfait

Ingredients

4 servings a recipe.

2 cups blueberries, fresh or perhaps thawed frozen

2 (eight ounces) cartons yellow yogurt

Ten gingersnaps

Preparation

In four bowls, wine glasses, and perhaps mason jars, set 1/4 cup blueberries, followed by 1/4 cup yogurt, and previously crumbled gingersnaps.

Duplicate to make two layers of each component

3. Easy Deviled Eggs

Ingredients

12 helpings a recipe.

12 large eggs

1/4 cup mayonnaise

One teaspoon yellow mustard

paprika for garnish

Preparation

Place eggs in a pot of water and get to a boil.

Boil the eggs until they are hard boiled; roughly 15 minutes.

Drain eggs and let cool.

Peel the egg shells as well as slice eggs half lengthwise.

Remove and mash together in a bowl, blending until crumbly.

Mix mayonnaise with mustard and yolks.

Spoon mixture into each white color of an egg as well as spread with paprika for color.

Place in the refrigerator to cool before serving.

4. Straightforward Pizza Sauce

Ingredients

12" Pizza helpings a recipe.

6 oz tomato paste

1-2 tablespoons olive oil

One teaspoon dried oregano

One teaspoon dried parsley

1-2 teaspoons fresh basil

2-3 tablespoons water

<u>Preparation</u>

Mix all components, including a little water, until you have a nice spreadable consistency.

Spread on top of 2 pizzas and add toppings.

5. Edamole Spread

<u>Ingredients</u>

6 (2 1/2 tablespoons each) servings per recipe.

3/4 cup frozen shelled green soybeans (edamame), thawed

Three tablespoons water

2 tablespoons olive oil

One tablespoon lemon rind, grated finely

1 tablespoon lemon juice

1/4 cup parsley leaves

1/4 teaspoon tabasco or hot sauce (optional)

One garlic clove halved

Preparation

Blend all ingredients, processing until smooth.

Cover and chill.

Serve with pita wedges or tortilla chips

6. Fajita Flavor Marinade

Ingredients

15 servings per recipe.

Juice from 2 limes

Juice from 1 orange

Juice from 1 grapefruit

3 tablespoons vegetable oil

One jalapeño, finely diced

Two cloves garlic teaspoon dried

Preparation

Mix all ingredients inside a small bowl.

Pour meat and vegetables on it to coat.

Soak for a minimum of one hour before grilling, pan-frying, or barbequing.

7. Great Fudge

<u>Ingredients</u>

48 servings per recipe.

32-ounce semi-sweet chocolate chips

4 (1 oz) squares unsweetened chocolate, chopped fine

 One teaspoon baking soda

2 (14 oz) cans sweetened condensed milk

2 tablespoons of vanilla

2 cups of walnuts

<u>Preparation</u>

Line bottom part of 9″×13″ pan with aluminum foil.

Spray with non-stick spray.

Toss chocolate and sodium bicarbonate on top of the double boiler until well blended.

Mix for condensed milk and vanilla.

Put over with a minimum of two cups.

Mix milk chocolate 2 to 4 minutes, with a spatula until it almost melts. A few small parts must be left.

Remove pan from heat and mix until milk chocolate is melted as well as the combination is smooth.

Mix in nuts.

Shift towards the pan.

Refrigerate for 2 hours, until ready.

Eliminate fudge from the pan.

Cut fudge into forty eight (one 1/4 inch) squares.

8. Quick Fajitas

<u>Ingredients</u>

4 (two fajitas each) servings a recipe

1 tablespoon olive oil

A carrot juice as well as the zest of lime

1 lemon zest and juice of orange or lemo

1 teaspoon cumin

Dash of cayenne pepper

1 pound meat, tofu, legumes, bite-size bits

1 onion, sliced

2 bell peppers

8 corn tortillas

Cream to taste

Cilantro to taste

Preparation

Combine oil cumin Cayenne pepper in a small bowl to help make the marinade.

Marinade and place vegetable meat in a tote Or maybe shallow dish and then marinate overnight

In a big skillet over medium high heat, cook Marinated beef, along with veggies until the onions start to be tender and start to caramelize (turn light brown), as well as the beef is cooked through. This should take no less than 15 20 minutes.

Drink tortillas and leading with sour cilantro and cream.

9. Brief Roast Chicken with Lemon & Herbs

Ingredients

3-ounce servings a recipe.

One (4 5 pounds) of entire chicken, fresh and thawed

2 tablespoons of unsalted butter softened

Two 1/2 tablespoons of chopped herbs that are fresh (sage, , thyme etc.)

2 cloves garlic, smashed as well as peeled

A little lemon, thinly sliced

One tablespoon olive oil

Preparation

Preheat oven to 450 degrees.

Place the chicken in a skillet.

Blend the herbs, butter, and garlic in a big bowl.

Place the butter within the body cavity of the chicken.

Rub the oil on the bird's skin.

Roast for fifteen minutes a pound, or perhaps until internal temperature reaches 165 degrees.

Drain the buttery pieces and juices of orange and put it over chicken.

Let chicken rest for twenty minutes before carving.

10. Ferocious Low Sodium Barbecue Sauce

Ingredients

Sixteen servings a recipe.

1 (six oz) low-salt tomato paste

1/4 (six ounces) water

1/4 cup black molasses

1/2 cup sautéed onion, minced

1/8 glass wine vinegar

2 tablespoons sugar

One tablespoon Worcestershire sauce

One tablespoon mustard

One teaspoon orange juice

One 1/2 teaspoon barbecue spice, consider our Salt Free BBQ Rub

Preparation

Blend all ingredients in a saucepan and stir over low heat fifteen minutes.

May require refrigeration for as much as fourteen days.

11. Sauteed Fresh Greens

Ingredients

2 servings a recipe.

4 cups of packed greens mustard, collard, kale or perhaps mixed

1 tablespoon of olive oil

1 glass of thinly sliced onion

1/4 teaspoon of ground turmeric

1/2 teaspoon sugar

1 tablespoon very low sodium soy sauce

1/2 cup of white rice or wine vinegar

1/4-1/2 teaspoon sesame seeds and sesame oil for garnish

Preparation

Cut greens into two″ extensive shreds.

Heat oil in a wok.

Sauté onion until translucent.

Sprinkle turmeric over onions.

Add cover and sugar.

Reduce heat and allow vapor within the juices of theirs till delicate. About 5-8 minutes. (During this time, uncover as well as turn sometimes. Add just a little water when sticking.)

With a slotted spoon, remove greens, making juices.

Add soy sauce as well as heat and wine to boil.

Eliminate once the sauce has thickened somewhat. Put the sauce over greens.

Garnish with sesame oil and seeds.

12. Watermelon Salsa

Ingredients

6 servings a recipe.

3 cups chopped, watermelon

1 cup green bell pepper, chopped

2 tablespoons lime juice

1 tablespoon cilantro, chopped

1 tablespoon green onion, chopped

2 moderate jalapeño, minced and seeded

A garlic clove, crushed

Preparation

Combine all ingredients, blend well.

Refrigerate for a minimum of one hour before serving.

This is wonderful for a dip or perhaps as a sauce for fish or chicken.

13. Flavorful and fragrant Basmati Rice

Ingredients

Eight servings a recipe.

One tablespoon unsalted butter

1/2 teaspoon ground turmeric

1/2 teaspoon ground coriander

1/2 teaspoon ground cardamom

One teaspoon garlic, minced

One cup of white-colored basmati rice

One 2/3 cups very low sodium chicken broth

Preparation

Heat butter in a big skillet over medium heat.

Add garlic and spices.

Sauté for one minute.

Include rice and mix until coated with spices and butter.

Include chicken broth.

Take to a boil, then reduce heat to medium low.

Simmer and cover for fifteen minutes.

14. Innovative Corn Salad with Sweet Chili Lime Sauce

Ingredients

4-6 servings a recipe.

Juice and zest of 2 limes

2-3 garlic cloves, minced

2-3 tablespoons Thai sweet chili sauce

Two cups corn kernels

A white onion, chopped

One lot cilantro

1/2 head white cabbage, shredded

1/2 cup shredded carrot

1/2 glass (chopped or even total) roasted, unsalted peanuts

Preparation

Combine lime juice, garlic, zest, and chocolate Sauce in a bowl.

Blend completely.

Blend veggies in a big bowl, drizzle dressing, and gently toss.

Chill or even serve immediately.

15. Fresh Fruit Lassi

Ingredients

Two servings a recipe.

One cup plain yogurt

1/2 glass milk

1/2 glass mango juice(or peach or perhaps apricot nectar)

1-3 teaspoon sugar to taste

1/4 teaspoon cardamon (optional)

1/2 teaspoon rose water (optional)

1/4 cup lime juice (optional)

Preparation

Place in a blender or food processor and blend for two minutes, then pour into specific function and glasses

16. Fresh Marinara Sauce

Ingredients

Sixteen servings a recipe.

15 moderate ripe tomatoes 6 pcs of garlic cloves, minced

2 pcs of big onions, chopped

3-4 pcs of big carrots, grated

1/3 cup olive oil

2 tablespoons dry looking or 1/3 glass fresh basil, chopped

One tablespoon dry looking or 3 tablespoons fresh oregano

One teaspoon pepper

Preparation

If working with fresh berries, set a couple in the water at a time

Raise it out there with a spoon and plunge in to the water.

Peel skins off and coarsely chop berries get 11 to 12 cups.

If using canned very low salt tomatoes, chop them too.

In a 5 quart or even larger container, place onion and carrots in oil over medium high heat, often stirring until onions are clear.

Include oregano, tomatoes, basil, and pepper.

Bring it to a boil, then lower the temperature and allow it to simmer. Stir often until the sauce has thickened. Serve over pasta.

Freeze sauce in food containers. Storage bags required.

17. Fried Apples

<u>Ingredients</u>

5 servings a recipe.

Five cups apples, chopped as well as peeled

Two teaspoons cinnamon

One teaspoon vanilla

<u>Preparation</u>

Spray skillet with nonstick covering.

Add apples.

Sauté apple.

Add cinnamon as well as vanilla.

18. Fruit & Herb Vinegars

<u>Ingredients</u>1-quart jar vinegar, white, like cider, white or red wine

1/2 glass berries or perhaps fresh fruit, cut into 1/2" bits

3-4 sprigs fresh herbs

Recycled classic salad dressing jars bottles

<u>Preparation</u>

Pour vinegar from the jar.

Clean and prepare the fruit. You need it to suit the jar, so chop parts of 1/2 inch. At the roof of the container, drop them for little fruits like blackberries or blueberries. Try some combination you like or even attempt Tarragon along with Italian Plum.

Blackberry Vinegar working with a vanilla bean is a mixture. For vinegar, garlic, or basil, thyme, attempt sage, and leek and tomato. Any kind of mixtures you can think of, try to keep the amount to roughly 1/2 glass of herbs and fruit a spoonful of vinegar.

Let sit at room temperature for 1 hour.

Strain vinegar by way of a cheesecloth bag or strainer.

Pour several natural fruits and herbs into jars.

Store at room temperature or even refrigerate for a season.

19. Fresh fruit Bars

<u>Ingredients</u>

Twenty four servings a recipe.

Two cups flour

1/2 glass sugar

One teaspoon baking powder

1/2 cup vegetable oil

One particular egg

1/4 glass water

One teaspoon vanilla extract

One glass jam (strawberry, raspberry, grape, blackberry)

<u>Preparation</u>

Preheat oven to 400 degrees.

Blend flour, baking powder, and glucose.

Stir oil.

Add egg, vanilla extract, water, and blend very well.

Press 2/3 of batter in a 9×9″ or maybe 8×8″ greased pan.

Spread with jam.

Make use of the remaining batter to make crumbs on top.

Bake for 25 or 30 minutes.

Cool in pan and cut in 24 bars.

20. Fresh fruit Julius

Ingredients

25-ounce servings Calories a recipe.

2 teaspoons tang powder

1/2 glass egg substitute

1/2 glass juice: orange, cranberry, grape or perhaps Additional

3 ice cubes

Preparation

Blend all Ingredients until smooth except ice.

Add ice; blend until slushy.

21. Fresh fruit Salsa

Ingredients

4 servings a recipe.

3/4 glass pineapple

3/4 cup mango, diced

1/2 cup strawberries, diced

1/4 cup white onion, diced

One jalapeño stemmed, seeded, and finely diced

Two tablespoons fresh mint leaves, chopped

Two tablespoons orange juice

One tablespoon lime juice

Preparation

In a ceramic bowl, blend the ingredients and mix to blend.

Cover with plastic wrap and permit salsa to marinade for aproximatly 20-30 minutes.

22. Fruit Vinegar Chicken

Ingredients

Six servings a recipe.

Two pounds of chicken

1/2 glass fruit or even berry vinegar

1/4 glass oil

1/4 cup orange juice

1/2 teaspoon marjoram

1/2 teaspoon basil

1/2 teaspoon tarragon

Preparation

Preheat oven to 350 degrees Celsius.

Combine all ingredients within a big zip lock bag.

Marinade for 15 to 20 minutes in the refrigerator.

Get rid of chicken out of the bag and put it in a baking dish.

Bake for roughly thirty minutes or perhaps until chicken gets to an internal temperature of 165 degrees.

23. Fruit Vinegar Salad Dressing

IngredientsTwo tablespoons sesame seeds

One tablespoon poppy seeds

Two tablespoons olive oil

1/4 glass fruit or even berry vinegar

2 tablespoons sugar

1/4 teaspoon paprika

1/3 glass green onions, thinly sliced

Preparation

Sesame seeds and heat poppy in oil until seeds are golden, for five minutes.

Cool.

Blend vinegar, sugar, and paprika until sugar dissolves.

Oil cooled with green onions and seeds.

Serve over salad.

24. Fruity Chicken Salad

<u>Ingredients</u>

8 servings a recipe.

Two cups chicken breasts, cubed prepared and 12.5 ounces might chicken

One cup sliced almonds

One stalk celery, chopped

A green onion, chopped

Two cups seedless grapes

An apple, cubed

3/4 glass raisins

1/2 cup sour cream

1/4 glass mayo

One teaspoon rice vinegar, unseasoned

Two teaspoon sugar

1/2 teaspoon Chinese Five-Spice Blend

Preparation

In a bowl, grapes, apples, Green onion, celery, almonds, combine chicken, and raisins.

In a bowl mix sour cream Rice vinegar, Oriental Five Spice Blend, and glucose.

Blend dressing to chicken mixture.

25. Gingerbread

Ingredients

One glass Master Mix

Two tablespoons sugar

1/4 teaspoon cinnamon

1/4 teaspoon ginger

1/4 teaspoon cloves

1 egg

1/4 glass molasses

1/4 glass water

Preparation

Preheat oven to 350 degrees.

Stir and combine spices.

Blend egg, water, and molasses.

Stir the mixture and beat for two minutes.

Stir in liquid and beat for one minute.

Bake in a skillet lined with wax paper for 40 minutes. Makes 4″×6″ cake.

CHAPTER 21

How To Be Successful On A Renal Diet

There is no specific renal diet, just tips that will help you control the levels of salt in your bloodstream through what you consume.

The diet necessary to counteract deficiency varies with each case, the harshness of the malfunction, whether the swelling is present, if you are over-weight, exactly what your blood electrolyte readings are, and if you are a candidate for dialysis or not.

With kidney failure, the salts in the bloodstream are thrown off balance. Diet guidelines aim to assist in controlling the build-up of waste products and fluid in your blood by putting less pressure on your system.

Renal diet plans are constructed around blood test results and a normal balanced diet that is healthy. The concept is to limit consumption. Fluids may be limited if your kidneys are unable to excrete sufficient water. So wastes like urea are kept at a minimum, protein intake is limited.he salts which commonly have to be limited are:

Sodium.

Sodium can cause blood fluid and pressure retention. Most renal diets use minimum salt in cooking, and stipulate, "No added salts." "Lo-salt" mixes aren't acceptable for salt replacement because they have high potassium levels, and shouldn't be used. Sausages, processed foods, sauces, ketchup, and canned foods must be avoided.

Phosphorus cannot be removed by dialysis so it may become an issue. Amounts are kept under control by medication and diet and are monitored. Phosphorus foods include dairy products, legumes, peas, beer, and cola drinks.

Potassium should be restricted if the blood levels are significant. Fruits and many vegetables contain potassium. High fiber foods include avocados, orange juice, bananas, apricots, beets, spinach.

Proteins are a necessary part of a wholesome diet and should only be consumed in tiny quantities. This includes all fish, poultry, eggs, and dairy products.

Fluids may be restricted if water retention is generalized swelling or fluid in the lungs. Fluids are strictly controlled for patients on hemodialysis. Fluids include water, soups, all beverages, and juices.

Carbohydrates are energy meals and should not be restricted unless you are diabetic or overweight. Lastly, it may be

advisable to take vitamins and vitamin supplements to enhance your immune system.

Following good diet guidelines will help slow down the reduction of kidney function and reduce the workload of the damaged kidneys. The renal diet guidelines are intended to help keep kidney victims healthy and functional to encourage and augment their therapy. It is very important to get specific advice from your physician and dietitian at all times.

CHAPTER 22

Diet Tips To Effectively Combat Renal Failure

Before dealing with the changes that are required to combat renal failure, it'll be helpful to understand that this illness isn't the only health criticism of the times. There are a couple of other complications like diabetes or heart disease that lay hidden in several patients for quite a while.

In such a scenario, a diet called the renal meal program is prescribed, including items that are low in carbohydrate content and high concerning the fat that was specially prepared. Additionally, such a specialized type of menu ensures that your body gets the ideal amount of nutrients that are necessary to be sure the road to healing is safe and steady.

In reality, these patients can hope to postpone dialysis for a while their bodies accomplish the changes and react positively. This should motivate you to continue with homemade remedies to address and heal renal failure in an ultimately effective method.

Some popular items that are prescribed for patients diagnosed with renal failure are:

A. Fruits like pineapple and berries such as cranberry, raspberry, blueberry and strawberry

B. Tea varieties such as Java tea and green tea

C. Herbal extracts from

• Rehmannia

• Cough bud

• Uva ursi

D. Items low in fat and protein

E. Grape seeds and seeds

What are the characteristics of a kidney diet?

Authentic to its growing popularity, this type of diet schedule is being advocated by dieticians and medical practitioners across the world. A couple of examples of an average day of this plan is something like:

A. Egg whites included and the yellow parts excluded

B. Lean red meat included and fat excluded

C. Fish but only certain varieties low in fat and in minimal quantities

D. Inclusion of carbohydrates, up to 8g per day

E. Fresh fruits like citrus ones as they contain less sugar and minimum fleshy content

F. The cereals, grains, and condiments included in your diet should be complete since they have a low-fat content

G. Berries such as asparagus, Onion, cabbage, celery, parsley, and sprouted kidney beans

H. Items made in flaxseed oil or flaxseed oil itself

Typically, within this kind of diet, there is a recommended diet program on a per-day foundation, which comprises various elements like magnesium, calcium, potassium, protein, fluids,

sodium, etc. The nature of these diet recommendations fluctuates based on the seriousness and the state of the failure of the renal system.

To reduce the burden on the kidneys, a renal diet is intended to function as an answer to those thinking about a way to reverse kidney disease. There are many advantages attached to the plan of meals as the patients can avoid developing some things related to kidney diseases, such as obesity and cardiovascular disease.

CONCLUSION

A renal diet is a highly nutritious one for patients with kidney issues. It is estimated that only 25 percent of the entire amount of nephrons are required to keep renal function. That usually means that the renal failure process is well protected from failure. It also suggests that at the time a patient has symptoms and signs of renal failure, kidney damage has occurred.

A dietary adjustment is necessary following things like the accumulation of waste products, impaired excretion of vitamin deficiencies electrolytes, and catabolism. Wasting syndrome is an issue. The customer with renal failure always loses body weight, muscle mass, and adipose tissue.

The objective of this renal diet is to keep a balance of electrolytes, minerals, and fluid in patients that are on dialysis. This is important because dialysis filters alone can't eliminate the wastes within the body. This is where a suitable diet comes in.

Dietary intake of electrolytes can be encouraged or restricted. The regulation of sodium is a delicate matter. Occasionally, sodium ingestion creeps in and a substitute must be found. However, the kidneys retain sodium.
Some consider that there ought to be a restriction as a principle of urinary sodium with observation. Another thing is the observation of status that gives essential information regarding sodium requirements.

Renal failure and its therapies significantly alter the quality of family life. There may be stressors and life changes. Much of the care required by clients receiving chronic peritoneal dialysis and hemodialysis and their significant others worry about the psychosocial aspects of dialysis.

This is not like every diet out there. It is a measured guide about how best to approach the symptoms and signs of renal failure. Also, it specifies the amount of fluid, electrolytes, minerals, and dietary protein which are allowable for each individual.

With the rampant spread of renal failure worldwide, it is understandable that a lot of renal diets have begun to sprout up. There are also many scam sites that claim to have a "quick fix renal diet," so be cautious. It is important to do your research and select sites that are genuine.

A balanced diet and exercise are recommended for everyone.. The demands of a diet are comprehensive and extensive to the person. A diabetic diet is suggested for many patients, but there aren't any one set diets for everybody.
The quantities and kinds of foods consumed will vary widely from person to person. The secret is to accommodate the renal diabetic diet to the patient's needs. To date diabetes cannot be cured, but it can be controlled via a well-managed diet.

Maintaining a healthy weight is vital for people with diabetes. A renal diabetic diet can help get the individual to that weight and help to keep it. Weight reduction or obesity will cause symptoms to worsen and lead to additional health problems with other organs and kidneys.

Consistent weight can also cause problems for the person with diabetes. When their weight keeps changing, having the ability to maintain the right amount of insulin within the body becomes difficult. A diabetic diet that is consistent supports the right quantity of insulin and helps level out these fluctuations.

Most foods can be eaten by people with diabetes, but depending on the type and the seriousness, it may be necessary to limit the amounts of specific foods. This list could consist of sugars, fats, and carbohydrates, particularly trans-fats.

Alcohol should be avoided, but may be consumed in small quantities and only on occasion. In general, the amount of the timing of foods and food consumed needs to be monitored. This is the key advantage of this esophageal diet

If you have been diagnosed with Diabetes, you have to work with a doctor and nutritionist to come up with a diet that is customized as soon as possible to get your condition in check. Diabetes is permanent. You won't outgrow it.

Even Type I, juvenile diabetes, won't be outgrown. Following a diet is the only way to handle this condition. Adult-onset, type II diabetes could be managed just by changing your diet. Adhering to a renal diet may be the answer.

Sometimes you'll need the diet and take oral drugs. Sometimes you'll need a renal diabetic diet and insulin injections. But no matter what your doctor recommends, be sure to adhere to the prescribed esophageal diet for your continued good health.

82993158R00110